GENERATION SLEEPLESS

GENERATION SLEEPLESS

Why Tweens and Teens Aren't Sleeping
Enough and How We Can Help Them

Foreword by Daniel J. Siegel, MD

Heather Turgeon, MFT, and Julie Wright, MFT

a TarcherPerigee book

an imprint of Penguin Random House LLC
penguinrandomhouse.com

Most TarcherPerigee books are available at special quantity discounts for bulk
purchase for sales promotions, premiums, fund-raising, and educational needs.
Special books or book excerpts also can be created to fit specific needs.
For details, write: SpecialMarkets@penguinrandomhouse.com.

Illustrations by Ben Hansford

Hardcover ISBN: 9780593192139
eBook ISBN: 9780593192146

Printed in the United States of America

1st Printing

Book design by Laura K. Corless

Contents

Foreword

If you are reading these words, you are awake. And if you are awake, the brain inside your skull is busy building up by-products of all the electrochemical energy streaming through the massively interwoven networks of neural systems that help us pay attention, be aware, remember, feel, think, and behave. Imagine what might happen if that accumulation of the day's leftover chemicals inside your head were not able to be cleaned up and removed. What a mess that would be! It would be as if you were the host of a party, passing out beverages and snacks, and were unable to clean up the celebratory garbage that remained.

Now imagine if that brain inside you was that of an adolescent. During this important period of brain remodeling, unused neural connections are being pruned away and, later on, enhancements in connectivity will be created by laying down a powerful sheath, myelin, to increase the speed and coordination of neural activity. This pruning and myelin formation are the basis of the important reconstruction process that characterizes our brain's busy growth process during the teen years and beyond, long into our twenties.

For proper brain function and growth to occur, the by-products of neural activity must be cleaned out on a regular basis. How does that cleaning occur? *During sleep.* Sleeping well and long enough to enable the "cleanup crew" of supportive glial cells to do their crucial detoxifying work is essential for teenagers to be able to effectively focus their attention, remember, think, make decisions, regulate their emotions, and interact with others. Sleep also is vital for teens to metabolize food well and prevent overeating, obesity, and the risk of illnesses such as diabetes. As if that were not enough to get us to hop into bed right now and catch some sleep, we also know that sleeping well and long enough reduces life-threatening systemic inflammation in our bodies.

Heather Turgeon and Julie Wright are the "sleep whisperers" who have created this science-backed, practical tip-packed guide to understanding sleep and creating a full and healthy life for our adolescents (and younger kids, as well as ourselves). Their work is not only creative and compelling, it is a contribution exactly when we need it—at a time when mental health challenges have never been higher. In modern times, not just during a viral pandemic, but simply in the VUCA times in which we live—VUCA being an acronym for the volatile, uncertain, complex, and ambiguous moment of contemporary cultural life—we are faced with social disconnection and unrest, emotional stress and worry, and internal processes of despair and confusion that make sleep even more a priority than ever. Add to this state of affairs the digital, electrically powered lives of social media that draw our social brains into states of feeling inadequate and left out, and leave our visually based brains activated with intense light at night when the brain is ready for sleep. Taken together, it's a prescription for disaster.

Generation Sleepless applies as much for adolescents in their important period of brain growth and remodeling as it does for us adults who care for teens, by using our mind's capacity to be resilient and collaborative. With huge numbers of youth getting inadequate amounts and quality of sleep, mental and medical health are compromised. With our minds unable to function at their optimum, we lose the ability to stay clear and focused in our attention, to think deeply about a problem we are trying to solve or a decision we need to make, and to remember the vital information we are learning at school and at home. Our relational lives suffer as well, as our emotions are set to threat mode and we can fly off the handle more easily and rupture our interpersonal connections. As adolescents are profoundly social beings, with being connected equated with survival, this relational friction can lead to more isolation and despair, impairing quality sleep with the ensuing stress of a life disconnected, and the cycle is in a downward spiral.

Enter our intrepid sleep whisperers. With compassion and creativity, Turgeon and Wright meet us where we are, understanding the challenges of modern adolescents and their parents, and offering practical strategies and accessible tools that can help us all gain the benefits of a good night's sleep. You'll learn in these powerful pages the science of sleeplessness, the benefits of good sleep, the ways in which schools and other entities that support teens can become "sleep-friendly," and the skills to change your life habits at home to make a more sleep-wise environment. Just imagine the benefits for us as parents to learn the fundamentals of sleep that empower us to make such a huge difference in our adolescents' lives now, and for decades to come. Yes, it's a practical dream come true, when sleep allows our creativity and memory consolidation to flourish. You have the choice right in front of you. Will you prioritize sleep for your teen just as you would their safety and health? The lessons to turn possibility into reality are here in this marvelous book. Think about this decision to honor the well-being of your family. Before you decide, you may simply want to sleep on it and enjoy the fruits of prioritizing sleep for everyone!

Daniel J. Siegel, MD

PART I

THE PERFECT STORM

1

The Great Sleep Recession

What if you knew that one simple daily habit would boost your teenager's mental health threefold, improve their grades and love of school, make them a better athlete, dramatically reduce their stress and anxiety, cut their chances of getting in a car accident in half, and ward off chronic health conditions like type 2 diabetes, obesity, and cancer? And what if this practice cost nothing and was completely natural? No downsides—only upsides to everything you care about in your teenager's life.

Of course you'd start today.

The irony is that we have this powerful panacea available to us at this very moment, and every day we systematically neglect it. Yes, you've guessed it. It's the life-fueling practice of sleep—and our teenagers are in the midst of the worst case of deprivation experienced by any population in history.

Modern-day teens are the most sleep-deprived group of any individuals the world has ever seen: while the majority of elementary school kids get the optimal amount of sleep on most nights, that number drops to about 30 percent by middle school, and by their senior year, only 5 percent of teens get optimal sleep on school nights. And the numbers keep slipping. In 2015, 58 percent more teenagers were severely sleep deprived than in 1991. A recent survey of sixty thousand American high school students measured how well teens are faring in terms of basic health recommendations for sleep, screen use, and exercise. Only 3 percent of girls and 7 percent of boys reached these targets.

As therapists and sleep specialists, we've watched this downward trend in teen sleep. A "perfect storm" (a concept we'll explore throughout this book) of shifting biology, academic pressure, early high school start times, and a misconception that sleep is dispensable rather than essential has been steadily chipping away at teen sleep. But while that storm has been brewing for decades, the explosion of technology has taken this storm to Category 5 hurricane levels. The smartphone is getting harder and harder to put down. Technology is ever more brilliant at keeping teens engaged and connected (teen sleep took a notable dip after 2011 as the smartphone gained popularity). Meanwhile, the academic load on students continues to increase and kids are being prepped for college applications when they've barely stopped playing tag on the playground. Like never before, teens' sleep is being stolen from all sides.

To make matters worse, adolescence is a stage of life when proper sleep is vital and game changing—to a degree that few of us fully appreciate. Books on baby sleep are stacked high on our bedside tables, because no one doubts the importance of sleep to a growing baby. But the truth is, a teenager's brain is going through an equally important stage of growth (with potentially more life-altering and consequential outcomes). Adolescence is an awe-inspiring and pivotal developmental phase, when the brain undergoes massive reorganization and growth, and much of that vital work happens *during sleep*. Missing sleep raises the risk of mental health issues, heightens teen stress at a neurochemical level, makes athletes more accident prone, and causes the brain's memory storage to malfunction, which short-circuits learning and academic success. When sleep is missing, the ripple effects on mental and physical health are tremendous and exponential.

Even when we as parents try to protect sleep, we often feel like our hands are tied. Yes, most of us know our teen should get to bed on time, but many of us feel frustrated and powerless because the factors that truly limit sleep—insidious technology, academic overload, and in some cases punishingly early high school start times—feel out of our control. What can we possibly do? (Who's up for joining us in breaking into the headquarters of Big Tech to change the algorithms that create increasingly addictive platforms and games? Or magically signing a bill to make middle and high schools across the world start no earlier than 8:30 a.m.?) In all seriousness, what are parents, teens, and the people who care about them supposed to do to protect growing teenage brains and bodies?

The answers are in this book. In the chapters ahead, we will help you regain what decades of science have shown as the mental and physical benefits of good sleep. Together, we will explore the wonders of the teenage brain, the surprising powers of healthy sleep, and the roadblocks to

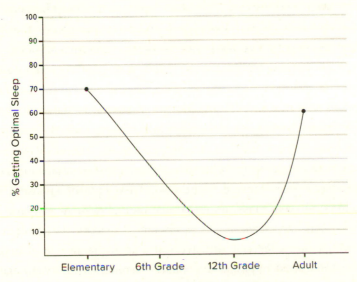

Sleep takes a nosedive during adolescence.

a teen's full night of slumber. We'll translate that knowledge into specific actionable steps that parents and teens—as well as school leaders, policy makers, and tech companies—can take right now to drastically transform sleep, and therefore health and well-being. We even have a "cheat sheet" for your teenager to read so they feel personally motivated to engage in these simple practices. And along the way, you'll find *yourself* engaging in better sleep—feeling healthier, happier, and more patient as well. (What can we say? It's never too late to start sleeping well.)

TEEN SLEEP LOSS: WHY IT MATTERS

Sleep breathes life into the adolescent brain—it releases neurochemicals like serotonin and dopamine that fuel teens with positivity, purpose, new ideas, passion, and sharp focus. It skyrockets hormones that strengthen and repair muscles. Sleep bolsters the immune system, decreases inflammation, and lowers the risk of chronic disease. If it seems like we could go on and on here, it's true. There is no drug, supplement, or routine that can return the same multifaceted benefits as good sleep.

And not surprisingly, the consequences of teenage sleep deprivation are serious and wide-reaching. Sleep loss creates wear and tear on the brain and body that manifests in many of the mental health symptoms we see in today's teenagers. According to the Pew Research Center, 7 in 10 teens say that anxiety and depression are major issues in their communities, and the number of teenagers who say they recently experienced depression increased 59 percent between 2007 and 2017. An increasing percentage of American youth say that they feel sad or hopeless, and tragically, the rate of suicide for adolescents increased nearly 60 percent between 2007 and 2018. Not coincidentally, during this time, sleep has continued to shrink. As we'll uncover in the next chapter, sleep loss raises stress levels, decreases the brain's emotional regulation pathways, and amplifies the brain's negative emotional centers. A sleep-deprived brain sees the world through a negative lens and skews toward sadness, frustration, anger, or hopelessness. A study of Chicago middle school kids found that those who got less sleep had lower self-esteem, lower grades, and higher levels of depression. One analysis found teens sleeping six to seven hours a night were 17 percent more likely to think about hurting themselves than those sleeping eight. Sleeping five hours or less made them 80 percent more likely. The connections between sleep and psychological well-being are direct and unmistakable. Mental health holds first place on every parent's concern list—which means sleep should too.

Lack of sleep dampens activity in the prefrontal region of the brain—where our judgment, decision-making, and self-regulation live—which means sleep-deprived adolescents are at higher risk for accidents and poor decision-making. This turns out to be especially dangerous for teen-agers, as we'll explain in chapter 2, because of the unique way the brain changes in these years. Car accidents, injuries, and many more terrifying and life-altering events that keep parents awake at night are exacerbated by sleep deprivation. Substance use goes up as sleep time goes down. In fact, data from the Centers for Disease Control and Prevention (CDC) links insufficient sleep to most risky behaviors, like smoking, drinking alcohol, sexual activity, lack of physical activity—along with seriously considering suicide. One study showed that each hour of lost sleep carried a 23 percent increase in the risk of tobacco, alcohol, or marijuana use, and a 58 percent increase in suicide attempts. Fatalities from car crashes are the leading cause of death among teenagers in the U.S., teen drivers are more than three times as likely as adults to be in a fatal crash, and sixteen- to twenty-four-year-olds constitute half of drowsy driving–related accidents (even though they make up significantly less of the driving population). Nearly 1 in 10 seniors in high school said they've fallen asleep while driving, and researchers have repeatedly estimated sleep deprivation as having similar effects to alcohol consumption. Sleep researcher Wendy Troxel points out that we'd never knowingly condone our teens drinking alcohol and getting behind the wheel, but without realizing it is a comparable risk, parents hand their keys to sleep-deprived teenagers all the time.

High schoolers burning the midnight oil, with their laptops open late at night, sacrifice hours of sleep to keep up with academic demands, but cramming facts while losing sleep turns out to be totally counterproductive. Sleep is needed to encode information and turn short-term memories into long-term ones. Without healthy sleep, the hippocampus, which is the region in the brain that encodes memories, essentially malfunctions, so students are unable to retain what they learned. Information goes in, but it doesn't stick. On the flip side, sleep improves focus and

SLEEP IS YOUR SECRET HEALTH WEAPON

Sleep is not rest. It's a vital activity with far-reaching health benefits. For example, sleeping well leads to healthy metabolism, eating behaviors, and weight—both now and in the future. Sleep regulates our body chemistry, which wards off future chronic health conditions like diabetes and heart disease. Cancer risk may even be affected by good sleep. Researchers injected mice with tumor cells under two conditions: one group was allowed normal sleep, while the other group had their sleep repeatedly disrupted. Mice whose sleep was disrupted had tumors twice the size as those who slept normally. Recently scientists have seen that sleep affects something called the glymphatic system in the brain, which is meant to eliminate toxins that have accumulated. When we sleep well, the brain's glymphatic system completes this important cleaning work.

Sleep is also crucial to the immune system. In a lab experiment, researchers gave the flu vaccine to severely sleep-restricted and well-rested students. The sleepy subjects produced 50 percent fewer antibodies than did the well-rested students.

attention, so well-slept kids absorb information better and are more likely to care about and enjoy what they're learning (which also helps them remember it later). Healthy sleep increases brain connectivity and decreases impulsivity and hyperactivity—meaning that kids who are considered to have behavioral issues are better helped by a full night's sleep than with a trip to the principal's office.

Many teens are so underslept on weekdays that they resemble subjects in acute sleep deprivation studies—falling asleep in class, seeing the world through negative eyes, forgetting information, making mistakes, and generally walking around in a cloud. Still more will suffer a lower level (thirty to sixty minutes) of chronic sleep loss that builds over time. In both cases, the effects are significant. Sleeping too little, or sleeping at the wrong times, as is the case for many teens whose internal clocks are out of sync with school schedules, sets off a cascade of chemical events in the body that affects the nervous system, raises stress hormones and blood pressure, increases inflammation, increases unhealthy eating, lowers testosterone and other important developmental hormones, and more.

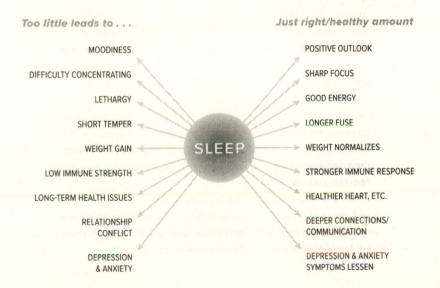

Too little leads to . . .

MOODINESS
DIFFICULTY CONCENTRATING
LETHARGY
SHORT TEMPER
WEIGHT GAIN
LOW IMMUNE STRENGTH
LONG-TERM HEALTH ISSUES
RELATIONSHIP CONFLICT
DEPRESSION & ANXIETY

SLEEP

Just right/healthy amount

POSITIVE OUTLOOK
SHARP FOCUS
GOOD ENERGY
LONGER FUSE
WEIGHT NORMALIZES
STRONGER IMMUNE RESPONSE
HEALTHIER HEART, ETC.
DEEPER CONNECTIONS/ COMMUNICATION
DEPRESSION & ANXIETY SYMPTOMS LESSEN

HOW MUCH SLEEP DO TEENS NEED, AND HOW MUCH ARE THEY GETTING?

How much sleep do you think adolescents need?

A. 6–7 hours
B. 7–8 hours
C. 9–10 hours

Most people answer B (although you may be onto us by now), when the answer is actually C. People tend to settle on B, because nine to ten hours sounds like how much sleep a young child needs. But here's a surprising notion: your teenager may need as much sleep now as he did in elementary school. This fact contradicts a widely held misconception we have about sleep—that kids need less of it as they grow. This turns out not to be true at all. Sleep needs for kids between the ages of ten and eighteen stay consistently high, and for many, this continues into early adulthood. Teens will sleep an average of 9.25 hours a night, if given the opportunity (a discovery that shocked scientists themselves, as we'll learn about in chapter 3), and in some cases they may need more sleep than their younger siblings.* Many people remark to us, "My teen sleeps all the time!" What they mean is that, when given the chance, on the weekend or on vacation, their teen sleeps extraordinarily long hours. This is the body attempting to make up for an accumulating backlog of sleep deprivation.

---

* For many teens, 8–8.5 hours is "adequate" and 9–10 hours "optimal." As with every age, teen sleep needs vary.

We underestimate sleep needs because we think of teens as near-adults. From a developing-brain perspective, they are not. In fact, teens are *beginning* a new wave of brain reorganization and psychological maturation that will last well into their twenties, and sleep is when much of this transformative construction happens. When adolescents sleep, neural pathways are refined and strengthened, emotions are processed, learned information and memories are encoded, muscles are repaired and grow, and many other systems in the body complete essential tasks. Adolescents have a deep need for sleep because of the magnitude of these changes.

Meanwhile, instead of nine to ten hours, the average twelfth grader in the U.S. sleeps 6.5 hours on a typical school night. The trend is stark. Many ten-year-olds tuck into bed early and have healthy sleep, but in middle school they start to lose their footing, and by the middle of high school they have fallen into severe sleep deprivation. By some estimates, kids lose about ninety minutes of sleep every night between sixth and twelfth grade—even though, during this time, their need for sleep does not go down. With so much missing sleep, the brain and body are taxed. During the week, most high schoolers are forced into an unnaturally early schedule and build up hours of "sleep debt"—or missing sleep that accumulates and can never be fully recovered. This is true even of teenagers who sleep seven to eight hours. On the weekend and holidays, kids desperately try to make up for lost sleep, forcing the brain's biological timekeeper into a lose-lose predicament through what we call "social jet lag." Social jet lag is the misalignment between the brain's clock and the outside world. A ninth grader recently told us that she's up on school days at 6:30 a.m. but sleeps until 10:30 a.m. when she has the chance—a common dilemma for teenagers as they struggle to pay back their sleep debt but confuse their brains in the process. As we'll see, this phenomenon of social jet lag is heightened in adolescence because of changes in the brain's sleep clock, and it comes at a significant physical and emotional cost. Aside from people like truck drivers and night-shift workers, this jet lag affects teens more than any other group of people.

Around the globe, adolescents are sleep deprived to varying degrees. A study in the *Korean Journal of Pediatrics* found that Korean high school

SLEEP INEQUITY

Children of color and families who live in disinvested communities are at higher risk for poor sleep, as well as sleep disorders. Sleep inequity is pervasive in the U.S. A study of middle and high schoolers found that non-white kids were more likely to be sleep deprived than their white counterparts, as were kids from families with lower household incomes. In a large sample of U.S. high school students, more than 1 in 5 Black students reported sleeping five or fewer hours per night. Studies from Canada, the U.S., Australia, and Norway have found that shorter and lower-quality sleep is more common in communities with fewer socioeconomic resources. In the U.S., this disparity in sleep health extends to adults as well, and may help explain other racial health disparities, as inadequate sleep contributes to higher rates of cardiovascular disease and other illnesses. Public health researchers and practitioners see this as an opportunity to address health disparities by supporting community sleep health.

Sleep loss may in part result from the stress of discrimination, as highlighted in recent research we'll look at in the next chapter. In addition, systemic racism's influence on neighborhood environment, access to physical activity amenities, constraints on work schedules and childcare, and stress overall pose challenges for families to sleep well. In chapter 5 we will see that kids who rely on public transportation are in particular taxed by long commute times that require waking up at unnaturally early hours.

The good news is that this means policies and initiatives that improve health care, reduce financial stress, and invest in a community's physical environment have the potential to improve sleep and, in turn, many other aspects of health.

kids, as a whole, were sleeping 5.7 hours a night, and most were falling asleep during the day. Another study of Korean students found that while fifth graders slept an average of eight hours on school nights, their sleep dwindled to six hours per night in tenth grade, 5.6 hours per night in eleventh grade, and a shocking 4.9 hours per night in the last year of high school. In South Korea, suicide is tragically the number one cause of death for adolescents. In Japan, 90 percent of adolescents have insufficient sleep. Teens in Germany fare better, sleeping 7.8 hours on school nights. Australian teens do particularly well, averaging roughly nine hours a night, and teens in Switzerland and Norway on average sleep more than eight hours, even on school nights. Adolescents in Belgium have been shown to get more than nine hours of sleep on school nights, and almost 10.5 on weekends.

In fact, given the concerning decline in teen sleep, the CDC—along with big-impact objectives like reducing deaths from drug overdoses and increasing access to safe drinking water around the world—has outlined "increasing the proportion of students in grades 9 to 12 who get sufficient sleep" as a global health priority.

UNTANGLING THE KNOT OF TEEN SLEEP DEPRIVATION: A TEAM EFFORT

Why are today's adolescents so sleep deprived? Answering this question is the first step to helping teens regain healthy sleep. As psychotherapists, sleep specialists, and moms ourselves, we've seen this perfect storm—or what we'd now call a hurricane—of factors converge to create a crisis of teen sleep deprivation:

We are not connecting the dots. When you consider the consequences of teen sleep deprivation, it seems shocking that we as a society haven't done something about it. But this is the hidden nature of sleep loss: we don't see it. We see anxiety and depression, ADHD symptoms, apathy, kids underperforming in school, or drug use. But even though sleep loss feeds all these issues, we don't connect the dots. In our therapy practice, we are constantly surprised by how little parents and teenagers complain directly about lack of sleep, or recognize it as a problem. They complain about irritability, injuries, school struggles, difficulty concentrating, depression, or lack of motivation (all signs of sleep deprivation), but not lack of sleep itself. If we suggested that clean drinking water and nutritious food were not important, we'd be laughed out of the building. But sleep is just as vital as these elements—we actually need it to survive. Studies of other mammals show that they will die from sleep deprivation in about the same time frame that they will die from food deprivation.

SLEEP AS A COMPETITIVE SPORTS EDGE

Researchers at Stanford tested the effects of good sleep on college basketball players. The athletes were put on a sleep regimen that had them spend ten hours in bed each night. Their free-throw and 3-point-shot percentages improved by almost 10 percent (anyone who knows basketball can tell you that's a make-or-break advantage), and their sprint time and reaction time improved. They reported improved overall ratings of physical and mental well-being during practices and games. Varsity tennis players' serving accuracy also significantly improved when they slept at least nine hours per night. LeBron James has repeatedly described how crucial his sleep is and attributes a lot of his recovery and injury prevention to his sleep regimen. He has joked that his trainer asks him every day, "How much did you sleep last night? Did you get your eight or nine hours?"

When we gather with other parents, we talk about how our kids' travel team is doing, or how musical theater is going. But after babyhood is over, have you ever heard another parent ask, "Hey, how's your kid sleeping?"

School leaders are also suffering from a lack of understanding and appreciation of teen sleep, which means it has been shuffled to the bottom of the priority list. Healthy teenage sleep is not supported by school schedules, environments, and policies. For example, the school clock is out of sync with the adolescent's natural body rhythms, which leads to shortened sleep, social jet lag, and a myriad of negative physical and mental health effects. Excessive homework is an issue in many high schools, which directly contributes to teens staying up too late (and forgetting the information they're supposed to retain in the long term).

> Even though almost 10 percent of twelfth graders said they have fallen asleep at the wheel, roughly one-third said their driver's education curriculum had no information about drowsy driving. (Although, who knows, maybe they were so tired they forgot hearing about it.)

Our sleep monitor is off. This brings us to another truth: we are often wildly off base when it comes to measuring our own family's sleep loss and the toll it's taking. One study in Australia found that the majority of teens had at least one indicator of a clinical sleep problem, but only 14 percent of parents recognized a sleep issue in their teen. A National Sleep Foundation survey on teens and sleep found that 9 out of 10 parents thought their teen got enough sleep at least a few nights a week, when the vast majority did not. In fact, teenagers themselves see the problem more clearly than their parents do: more than half of teens said they know they don't get enough sleep and were too sleepy during the day. One survey found that only 35 percent of parents of fifteen- to seventeen-year-olds thought they needed nine hours or more. Many of our clients say they assume nine hours of sleep is a luxury for a teen rather than something that's essential for well-being and development.

SIGNS OF A SLEEP-DEPRIVED TEEN

- Has trouble waking up in the morning for school more than once a week
- Sleeps two hours longer or more on the weekend or vacations
- Falls asleep while studying, watching a movie, or during other passive entertainment
- Can fall asleep during the morning hours if given the chance (for example, on the way to school or in a morning class)
- Exhibits low energy, moodiness, irritability
- Shows lack of interest in school, boredom, or aimlessness
- Drinks caffeinated beverages or vapes (contains nicotine)
- Has no downtime or breaks, is overcommitted and overscheduled
- Takes late-afternoon or evening naps

As a society, we have accepted too little sleep as an inevitable part of growing up. We think it's normal that teens struggle to wake up in the morning and that many leave for school before the sun comes up. Our societal view of adolescents is that they can be moody, lazy, or rebellious or make poor decisions—which, oddly enough, are all classic signs of sleep loss. We puzzle over how to support them, all while ignoring this load-bearing pillar in their foundation of well-being.

The teen biological clock shifts later. Did you know that adolescents have unique biological clocks controlling the timing of their sleep and alertness? In the adolescent years, the timing of sleep changes at a neurological level. This change begins for most kids in middle school and remains with them until early adulthood. In these years, the brain's sleep clock is delayed, which makes adolescents naturally stay awake later at night and want to sleep later in the morning. It's not possible for most

ADOLESCENTS STRUGGLE TO STAY AWAKE

In the U.S., two-thirds of high schoolers have consumed energy drinks, which contain caffeine and the stimulant taurine and other chemicals. It's no surprise, then, that energy-drink-related ER visits increased tenfold between 2005 and 2011. In many European Union countries, including Germany and the UK, there has been a rapid expansion of the energy drink market to adolescents, with a recent survey finding that the majority of high school students had consumed them, and about a third did so on a regular basis.

The prevalence of adolescents vaping—often products containing nicotine, which is a stimulant—continues to go up. Monitoring the Future, a large U.S. study that has been tracking teen drug and alcohol use since 1975, has found that the increases in teen vaping have been the steepest of any substance recorded. As of 2020, a quarter of eighth graders had vaped, and half of twelfth graders. Vaping nicotine products doubled just between 2017 and 2019.

teens to just "go to bed early"—many cannot fall asleep until 10:00 or 11:00 p.m. no matter what they do. By the same token, the brain clock is programmed to be sleeping until closer to 8:00 a.m. Contrary to negative stereotypes, this has nothing to do with laziness. Waking at 6:00 a.m. means waking during a teen's "night" and missing hours of sleep.

And in a further plot twist, as we'll explain in chapter 3, teenagers are especially sensitive to environmental cues like light and technology. Their brains are more easily tricked to stay up later, and their sleep chemistry is more easily suppressed. This means proper sleep environments, routines, and timing are extra important for teenagers.

"TXT me, I'm only sleeping." There is a lot of scientific inquiry and discussion about how technology impacts sleep, which we will explore in chapter 4, but let's be clear: technology is a major force diminishing our

teenagers' sleep. Smartphones, video games, and social media steal sleep through multiple routes—which is why research shows a clear link between screen use and lower quality and quantity of sleep. In fact, sleep quality and adolescent mental health have both followed a downward trend as the saturation of smartphones has increased since 2010. As parents, we wouldn't let our kids go to bed sipping a venti cappuccino, but the majority of teens retire to their bedrooms with devices that have equal sleep-stealing powers. Most teens sleep with their phones at arm's reach—we talk to many who share a pillow with theirs—and parents tell us they feel they've lost control over screens and sleep hygiene. Technology companies, social media platforms, and so forth have captured our kids' attention and diminished their sleep, without having to take any responsibility for the consequences. Often, we hear the sentiment that there's nothing we can do about managing technology or keeping it out of the bedroom—Pandora's box is already open. But this is a myth. You have the ability to talk about this and make changes as a family, and it's revolutionary for sleep. We know how tricky this is because we're moms ourselves, but it's a needle we will help you thread. Within the home, empowering both teens and parents, understanding exactly how electronic media affects sleep, and changing habits (starting with parents' behavior) are some of the most powerful steps families can take. Within one week, these can transform sleep (not to mention improve family connection).

Early school start times and academic onslaught. By high school, a teen's sleep is encroached on from both sides. Excessive homework, technology, and delayed sleep chemistry push bedtimes later, while biologically unfriendly—in some cases downright abusive—school start times have some adolescents leaving the house before the sun comes up. Early high school start times are the norm in the U.S.—despite decades of evidence that they are harmful and pleas from parents, students, the American Academy of Pediatrics (AAP), and many others. At a developmental time when teens need more sleep, they are instead squeezed into the worst sleep crisis experienced by any age group. We all have a role to play: parents, teachers, principals, superintendents, sports coaches, and university admissions committees. Instead of working as a team to help and take care of teenagers, we ignore their basic need for sleep. Three hours of homework, mixed with baseball practice or dance rehearsals, a part-time job (all while technology hunts down their attention), and a 7:45 a.m. high school start time? Without change, the only mathematical outcome is massive sleep deprivation.

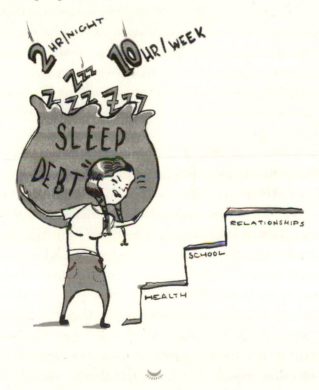

HOW TO REGAIN TEENAGE SLEEP

When you consider all the factors stealing an adolescent's sleep, it can seem like you're staring at an unsolvable math problem. Even though the stakes are high and the importance of good sleep is clear, the deck is truly stacked against adolescents sleeping well.

The good news is that problem is solvable. All the forces contributing to teen sleep loss are precisely the opportunities for reclaiming healthy sleep. While some of these forces require societal shifts, many of them force you, as parents and teens, have direct and immediate control over. When it comes to shifting habits at home, small changes make a big difference; even adding thirty minutes of sleep to your schedule wins you 2.5 hours of sleep by the end of the school week. And you have a simple and powerful truth on your side: sleep is natural, and our brains and bodies are programmed to do it. Sleep is observed in all animals, and it is vital and innate. With the adaptations we'll teach you in this book, sleep takes over, because, like thirst, hunger, and breathing, sleep is an organic drive. Over and over, we see this in our work: when we identify the factors stealing sleep and comprehensively help families to create new habits, sleep improves dramatically and quickly. This is not magic (although sleeping well feels magical); this is biology.

Open eyes to shut-eye. In the next two chapters, we will take a look inside the unique sleep needs and brain clocks of teens. Understanding how much sleep teenagers need and how their biology leads to a night owl proclivity will show us how to support better sleep habits. Teens will learn about their own sleep clocks, how their sleep affects what is important to them, and how to use this information to set habits and schedules for healthy sleep. In chapter 4, we'll learn how and why smartphones, social media, and electronic lights and devices impact adolescents' sleep so strongly. As we'll see in chapter 5, kids who have healthy school start times and sleep well can think clearly, critically, and creatively. They manage time, retain information, and, not surprisingly, do better in school. School administrators will find suggestions throughout chapter 5 for "sleep-forward" schools. Teams and schools will learn how they can harness the power of sleep to improve athletic performance, enjoyment, and academics.

Paleo-sleep. Sleep is natural, but the modern world is not. The human brain and the sleep clock within are constantly confused by the signals of modern life, and misaligned with the cues of the natural world. Our sensory systems, and especially those of teenagers, become out of sync when signals of light and activity occur at the wrong times, and this creates very late bedtimes, sleep loss, and social jet lag. The beauty is that you can use this information to change your habits and bring yourself more in line with the natural environment. Working with our bodies' natural sleep systems is what we call "paleo-sleep." You cannot avoid modern life (although we'll describe camping experiments that will make you want to buy your family a tent and leave the devices behind), but you can take control and manage it in a smart way that brings you more in sync with your natural sleep.

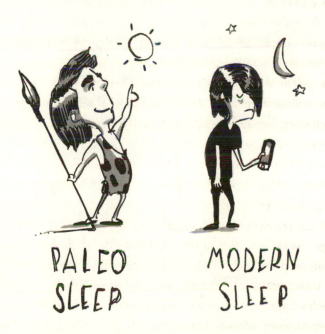

PALEO SLEEP   MODERN SLEEP

Our brains evolved to take cues from sun and darkness.
Modern life has disconnected us and reduces our sleep.

The Five Habits of Happy Sleepers. In chapter 6, you will learn the Five Habits of Happy Sleepers, which are actionable steps you and your family can take to significantly improve your sleep. With these habits in place, you create what we call the "sleep bubble." The sleep bubble is protective, allowing our sleep to self-regulate, and our brains and bodies to fill up on sleep, repair muscles, strengthen the immune system, consolidate memories, and more. When we adopt these habits, our mood improves, we have more interest in activities, we perform better in sports, we are more fun to be around, we write better papers. We feel like our best selves.

The habits you will learn in chapter 6 harness the power of physical and psychological practices and steps to improve the quality and duration of sleep. However, if teens suffer from more entrenched and resistant insomnia, then clinical treatment (often cognitive behavioral therapy for insomnia) is indicated. In this case, it's important to talk to a doctor or therapist who specializes in sleep.

Teen self-motivation. No surprise to any of us parents: a teen has to feel *motivated* to get more sleep; otherwise it won't happen. We will give you ample reasons for getting better sleep, but it's critical for teens themselves to connect the dots between how they feel, what they care about, and how sleep will support this. There are many examples of dialogue and ways to engage your teen throughout this book. No teenager wants to be told what to do, but in our experience, all teenagers like to feel healthy and happy. Teenagers need us to lead with empathy, listen to their ideas and priorities, give them information, have family conversations about sleep, school, and schedules, and gradually hand over control of such things to them as they grow. Teenagers have to find their own motivation for sleeping well. In chapter 8, we will teach you our three-step approach for empathic and effective communication so you have a place to start this dialogue. On page 225 you'll find suggestions for increasing motivation, and on page 188 you'll find a teen cheat sheet for better sleep.

Sleep forward. At the end of the day—when the stars come out and, hopefully, you're in your jammies climbing into your cozy bed—healthy sleep has to go beyond simple habits or checklists; otherwise the changes won't stick. Good sleep for a lifetime requires a shift in how we think about and prioritize the practice of sleep in the first place. Unfortunately, many families have been cornered into a *sleep-comes-last* approach, in which sleep is seen as dispensable, and is simply what is left after all the other priorities are met. This makes it easy to jettison thirty minutes or more of sleep, and over time, is why this sleep debt piles up. We will help you shift to a *sleep-forward* approach, which moves sleep from the back seat, holds sleep as a priority, sees it as essential, and organizes life around this priority. The sleep-forward approach can be adopted by parents, teens, high schools, sports teams, school districts, and more.

Many parents of teens tell us they've lost control over sleep routines. At age eight, kids have regular early bedtimes, book reading, a nightly chat, blanket tucking, and stuffed animals accompanying them to bed. Around age twelve, these sweet rituals begin to fade as parents figure kids don't need as much fanfare. By age fifteen, most kids go to bed later than their parents, do not read for pleasure, and share a pillow with their phones. Parents admit to us all the time that they've given up. They have no idea what time their children go to bed or how much they actually sleep. Phones, computers, and video games are in the bedroom, and the combination of schoolwork, extracurricular activities, and social and screen time creates an impossible math; sleep loses out. The truth is, though, that family habits are powerful, and research and clinical experience tell us that parental involvement does work, leading to better sleep and better health. A study of seventh graders found that the greatest predictors of an adolescent's sleep quality were the family sleep habits, such as having a regular bedtime, having sufficient wind-down time, and limiting screen exposure and caffeine before bed. In large, nationally representative U.S. samples, researchers see that adolescents with parent-set, earlier bedtimes had the best indicators of positive mental health. In this book, we'll help you find the right, age-appropriate level of involvement—especially using the concepts in chapter 7. And if you feel discouraged, remember that even thirty minutes more sleep every night is significant and potentially life changing.

As parents, teachers, coaches, mental health providers, education leaders, and anyone who works with and cares for teens, we all need to make healthy sleep a priority in order to see its positive ripple effects benefit our homes, schools, and society.

The time to protect and reclaim teen sleep is now.

HOW TO USE THIS BOOK

Part 1 of this book explores the teenage brain and the dazzling powers of teenage sleep. It also busts some common teen myths and will help you see behind the scenes, for some serious aha moments, a deeper understanding, and a boost of motivation. We dive deep into the science of teenage sleep and the unbelievable upsides of sleep, and we explain the circadian clock, along with why your teen may need extra prodding to get out of bed on Monday mornings. Chapters 4 and 5 examine what we consider the two biggest roadblocks to a teenager's full night's sleep: screens and school.

Part 2 is where we'll lay out the tools, habits, and practices, within your home, that you can implement to improve your teenager's sleep—tonight. The two parts of the book are symbiotic; they complement each other. With the level of understanding you get from Part 1, you'll be informed and inspired to begin your journey to better sleep for your teen.

2

The Essential Nutrient of the Adolescent Brain

L et's pause on talking about sleep for just a moment.

For now, we want to tell you about a miracle drug we've recently learned about. Derived from the outer layer of the "erom" plant, these erom peels have enormous benefits for teens, in multiple facets of life. This drug is known to improve focus and grades. It leads to a greater secretion of growth hormones and boosts the immune system, and aids with muscle repair. It lowers the risk of chronic conditions later in life, like cancer and diabetes. When teens take it, the frontal lobes of the brain become highly activated, so they enjoy school more and experience greater creativity. It increases the flow of euphoric neurochemicals in the brain, which lowers the incidence of arguments over homework, and has been clinically proven to reduce eye rolling. It decreases stress, increases positive mood, and makes adolescents open up and talk. In fact, *erom peels* may be the cure-all pharmaceutical of the future.

Okay, you're onto us already: spelled backward, *sleep more*. (What can we say—we're sleep experts, not comedy writers.) But can you see how, when described as a drug, sleeping more sounds too good to be true? There is no other naturally occurring daily practice in life that has such wide-reaching, dramatic, and versatile benefits as sleep.

Do you know when sleep is especially important? When kids are growing. Just as babies sleep inordinately long hours to feed their rapid brain growth, adolescents need high doses of sleep to feed a metamorphic period of brain development. This is why we'll take a moment to lay out some of the key changes in the fascinating teen brain. If biology wasn't your favorite class, it's okay; you'll quickly see how "aha" this information is. We'll upend some classic teen stereotypes, show you where sleep is pivotal, and help you feel inspired by your teen's magnificent developmental feats.

During adolescence, the brain undergoes massive and permanent restructuring. In this finale of brain development, the neural pathways in the frontal lobes, and in particular the prefrontal cortex—the hub of our wisdom, smart decision-making, emotional regulation, empathy, and judgment—become stronger and highly efficient. The brain cells in this sensible prefrontal region reach their connections down into the lower brain, where areas such as the limbic system, which includes our emotional generator, the amygdala, are. This means thinking and oversight areas of the brain are now more closely integrated with emotion and impulse areas of the brain. Psychiatrist Dan Siegel refers to this as connecting the "upstairs" and "downstairs" brain. As this happens, adolescents get better at planning, putting themselves in others' shoes, and balancing their feelings.

Guess when this transformative brain building happens? You got it: during sleep. The strengthening and refining of network connections throughout the adolescent brain occur during *sleep*—an aspect of life that many of us, and especially teenagers, are shrinking to dangerously low levels. In fact, sleep is so essential to brain development that researchers have asked the very legitimate question of whether sleep deprivation during adolescence may permanently alter the developmental trajectory of the brain and behavior. Many believe the answer is yes.

SLEEPING TO GROW

Recently, Heather's young adolescent son woke up after eleven hours of sleep, and she looked at him and remarked that he seemed taller. It wasn't a joke. He had actually grown (although, okay, maybe just slightly in perceptible height), but his brain had strengthened connections, balanced emotions (he woke up happy), and become more proficient at the skills he had practiced the day before. He was pulled into this long, deep night of sleep so he could get stronger, smarter, and faster (and yes, a little bit taller). In fact, across many species, from zebra fish to mammals, growing increases our need for sleep. In humans, this is because sleep is when we do the heavy lifting of building and refining the brain and body. Deep sleep is vital to the adolescent brain for many reasons, including the process of pruning, in which unused neural connections die off while others strengthen. The pruning process makes the adolescent brain highly specialized, integrated, and fast. In fact, sleep scientists have seen that deep sleep seems to intensify *before* a skill emerges—meaning that sleep isn't just recovery and rest, it's active construction. A recent study found that adolescents who had shorter sleep, later sleep timing, and poorer-quality sleep were more likely to have a thinner cortex (which is the highly complex, outermost layer of the brain).

This "remodeling" makes adolescence a sensitive period of development. The process of connecting the upstairs and downstairs brain and of pruning create amazingly wonderful explosions of creativity, exuberance, adventure, and possibility. This makes adolescence a period that is literally bursting with potential. It also makes it a vulnerable time, which is why adolescents are the most likely of all of us to develop mental health issues or to be in a fatal or life-altering accident. Our goal as parents, and as a society, is to feed the adolescent brain with healthy sleep so that kids come through this transformative period of their lives and flourish.

SLEEP PROTECTS AND NURTURES THE TEENAGE BRAIN

Sleep bolsters every aspect of an adolescent's life. But there are a few reasons that healthy sleep becomes crucial in these years:

SLEEP BOOSTS MENTAL HEALTH

The connections between sleep and mental health can and do fill entire books. It's a complex relationship. Where lack of sleep was once thought of as a side effect of mental and physical health conditions, we now know it can trigger, or at least exacerbate, them. An estimated 90 percent of children with depression experience sleep problems. Long-term studies of young people have found that sleep disruptions often *precede* mental health issues; in fact, in young people, sleep problems have been used to predict later depression and are considered a risk indicator. In other words, children with poor sleep are at greater risk of developing depression. A lab study of young people with an anxiety disorder found that they took longer to fall asleep and slept less deeply when compared to those without anxiety. Sleep issues are commonly associated with anxiety, depression, bipolar disorder, and ADHD. In fact, almost all mental health issues are connected with disrupted sleep. The results from the Youth Risk Behavior Survey (YRBS)—a large, nationally representative sample of high school students around the U.S.—found a significant link between poor sleep, mood, and self-harm. Kids who said they slept less than six hours a night were three times as likely as those who slept eight hours or more to say they had contemplated suicide.

Mental health is a critical issue in the adolescent years—in fact, many parents and doctors would say it's *the* issue. Adolescents are more vulnerable to stress, and most psychiatric disorders present themselves during the adolescent years. For parents, protecting kids' mental health and happiness by far feels like our most important priority.

ADOLESCENCE VERSUS PUBERTY

What is the difference between these terms? Puberty is a sequence of distinct physical changes that are caused by the brain and the release of hormones, with an average onset around ages eleven to twelve. Adolescence is a broader term for the phase of life in between childhood and adulthood, spanning approximately ages ten to twenty-five. It includes the body changes of puberty, but it also includes the changes we experience in our identity, relationships, emotions, and view of the world.

Sleep more, stress less

Healthy sleep feeds happy adolescents. There are many reasons for this. For one, proper sleep puts a positive filter on life. The flip side of this phenomenon was shown when researchers restricted the sleep of adolescents and adults to between five and 6.5 hours for a few nights, and then allowed them to have two nights of "recovery" sleep of 8.5 hours. When sleep deprived, all groups felt less "interested, excited, happy, energetic, cheerful, proud." The sleep deprivation particularly heightened the worries of the younger adolescents—they viewed their most worrisome item in life as significantly more threatening when sleep deprived. The authors interpreted this to mean young adolescents may be extra vulnerable to elevated anxiety when sleep deprived.

We all know that our mood and optimism darken without good sleep. The brain basis for this is unfolding in research labs, but it seems that sleep allows the higher regions of the brain to soothe, influence, and control the lower emotional brain regions (as we described, this upstairs-downstairs relationship is under remodeling in the teen years). When we don't sleep, the sensible higher brain is no longer as engaged, and the raw emotional brain, where fear, anger, and other reactive or negative emotions are generated, is left to fend for itself. Berkeley sleep scientist Matthew Walker conducted a lab experiment looking at this phenomenon, in which a group of young adults were sleep deprived for a day and a half, and then their brains were scanned as they looked at pictures of varying emotional states. In the sleep-deprived group, the amygdala (in the limbic, emotional center) was 60 percent more activated and had a threefold increase in volume over the control group, who had slept normally. The researchers called this a hyper-limbic response by the amygdala. There was also significantly weaker connectivity between the amygdala and

YOUTH VIOLENCE

Youth violence is a leading cause of injury and death for adolescents, and of course can have a devastating impact on communities and larger society. According to the CDC, youth violence results in more than 400,000 nonfatal injuries every year. Violent behavior is complex and difficult to understand or predict, but we do know that healthy sleep lowers risk-taking and poor decision-making, and helps us feel more optimistic and less reactive. Sleep is one piece of the puzzle when it comes to lowering the incidence of violent behaviors that have a wide-reaching impact on society.

the prefrontal cortex (again, upstairs-downstairs connection failure) than in the rested group. The implication here is that without proper sleep, the emotional centers of the brain may be overactive, and less comforted by the higher regulation centers. The researchers described this as a "failure of top-down, prefrontal control."

The data on mental health and sleep is vast. High school students with lower sleep times (7.5 hours) have higher levels of perceived stress than students with greater sleep times (9.7 hours). A study of high school seniors in New Jersey found that those who were very sleep deprived (which was many, as the average sleep time was 6.1 hours) were three times as likely to report strong symptoms of depression. The authors say point-blank that "sleep deprivation and depression go hand in hand in teenagers," and that instead of giving them medications, we should give them a chance to sleep. Particularly concerning for parents are findings showing that depression and suicidal ideation are associated with not just short sleep duration but also later or nonexistent bedtimes. In a study of more than fifteen thousand adolescents in grades 7 to 12, those with bedtimes set by parents of midnight or later were 24 percent more likely to suffer from depression and 20 percent more likely to have suicidal ideation than adolescents with parental-set bedtimes of 10:00 p.m. or earlier.

A recent study of Asian, Latinx, and Black adolescents illuminates one reason students of color are more likely to experience sleep issues. Fordham researcher Tiffany Yip had adolescents track experiences of discrimination over a period of four years, while also tracking sleep and other health symptoms. On days in which kids experienced discrimination stress, they had disturbed sleep that evening and greater sleepiness and daytime dysfunction the next day. The stronger the impact of this stress on sleep, the more likely kids were to have anxious or depressive symptoms in the longer term. This illuminates one route through which discrimination leads to a decrease in sleep, and a negative impact on an adolescent's well-being.

People of all ages are negatively impacted by sleep loss, but adolescents uniquely so, because of how the brain is remodeling, and because of the mental and physical consequences. Sleep is integral to teen mental health—balancing emotions, processing the day's experiences, and creating the optimistic beat we want them to hear as they approach every day. Considering sleep's role in mental health, when we hear that high school students are sleeping six or seven hours a night, our alarm bells should be going off.

SLEEP KEEPS ADOLESCENTS SAFE

Less sleep has repeatedly been linked to risky adolescent behaviors. In a recent example of this, Harvard researchers analyzed data from the YRBS and found that adolescents who report sleeping less than eight hours a night were more likely to drink alcohol, smoke and use other drugs, engage in risky driving behaviors, engage in risky sexual behaviors, and exhibit aggressive behaviors. Studies of adolescents in various countries show similar patterns: In Finnish adolescents, tiredness and poor sleep habits have been highly linked to substance use. Italian adolescents who don't sleep well were found to be more likely to smoke and drink alcohol than good sleepers.

Why exactly does sleeping less lead to unhealthy behaviors? The truth is that people of all ages make questionable decisions when sleep deprived. When we lose sleep, our higher powers of reasoning and impulse control (housed in the prefrontal cortex) are compromised. Little kids who sleep less have more tantrums, behavioral issues, and lower impulse control. Adults who sleep less make unhealthy food choices, and so forth.

The problem is that adolescents are already prone to risky decisions because of how the brain is transforming in these years. The dopamine system in the adolescent brain radiates more intensely. Most of us know dopamine as a chemical that gives us a strong feeling of positivity and reward and makes us want to do something again. But it also leads us to thrill seeking and is connected to addictive behaviors. In adolescence, we have an increased release of and sensitivity to dopamine. Brain imaging studies have shown that the nucleus accumbens—a brain region in the limbic system (in the downstairs brain)—peaks in sensitivity during mid-adolescence (around ages fifteen to sixteen). This area of the brain sends us strong driving signals to do something for a reward, without running it by the upstairs brain. This means that adolescents feel rewards intensely. The amount of sheer pleasure we get from something is high during adolescence, which makes our urges to do the most fun, enticing, and exciting activities at their peak. The whole brain is under the influence of dopamine, because projections or pathways that use it reach throughout.

This reward sensitivity shows a curved pattern, peaking in mid-adolescence, whereas impulse control slowly increases over time. Where the reward sensitivity outpaces impulse control may be a particularly dangerous period for some kids. Dopamine acts intensely on systems in the brain that both feel reward and anticipate reward, which is part of why adolescents are more prone to risky behaviors and also addictions. The control centers of the prefrontal brain regions, which strengthen through adolescence, can help kids make healthy choices. But with poor sleep, these control centers are essentially offline.

Risk and the adolescent "social brain"

No surprise to any of us, teenagers make different decisions when together versus when alone. For example, teens are more likely to be in a car crash when a fellow teen is in the passenger seat, whereas this is not true of adults. (This can also be seen in driving simulation studies, where teens take more risks when a peer is present, whereas adults do not.) The interesting part about this is that adolescents appear to be more sensitive and attuned to emotional information, in general, than little kids and adults, and this can be seen at the level of the brain. A team at Yale tested children, teens, and adults on a computer task that requires self-control—participants had to push a button or resist pushing a button when they were presented with images of different people's positive, negative, and neutral facial expressions. With neutral expressions, the adolescents scored as well or better than adults. When they saw happy, excited faces, though, the adolescents' self-control got worse and they made more errors (kids' and adults' performance stayed the same). As the participants were trying to perform this impulse control task while seeing emotional faces, an area of the brain called the "ventral striatum"— involved in detecting new and rewarding cues from the environment— was firing more strongly for the teens.

This and other brain research suggest a heavy social influence over the adolescent brain. In calm, nonsocial moments, teens often make coolheaded decisions, but with emotional information or peer influence, they are more likely to be swayed. This means that, in a sense, teens are more empathic than we are. But this can also cause teens to lose their moral compass and be influenced by other people and their feelings.

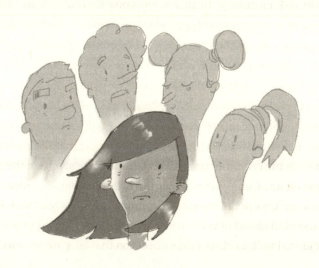

"Peer pressure" has more aptly been termed simply "peer presence," as it's not necessary for friends to actively put pressure on a teenager in order to sway the teen's moral compass. This actually makes good evolutionary sense, as humans are inherently social creatures and adolescence is a time of life when finding and identifying with peer groups is really important. The truth, though, is that the influence of peer presence can go many ways. Having positive peers who make good choices themselves is ideal for this reason.

Risk and the "invincibility" myth

People often say that teens feel invincible, and this is why they sometimes make bad choices. This turns out not to be true (another teen stereotype science does not support). Research indicates that adolescents are actually well aware of risks. They do think ahead, and they do assess the potential downsides. They know bad things happen.

So why would a teen be more likely than an adult to binge drink and go swimming in the middle of the night, or drive 100 miles an hour on a narrow highway? The answer seems, in part, that adolescents use a different risk calculator to make decisions than do adults. The reward and gratification from a certain behavior (thanks to the hyperactive dopamine system) are weighed more heavily than the potential negative outcome.

Think about this: For many risky or "irresponsible" behaviors, the probability of a negative outcome—like drowning in a pool or crashing a car—is technically low. In each instance, it's more likely it'll turn out okay than go wrong. So a high reward drive and low risk assessment leads to "Let's do it!" In fact, just thinking about a gratifying activity activates pleasure centers in the brain and releases dopamine, focusing us on the gratification or payoff itself, and overshadowing a bad outcome. This means that, as adolescents, we're not necessarily impulsive—we often think *hyperrationally* and plan ahead of time to get the desired reward—but we might still decide to break a rule or make a decision that later we see was less than wise.

Researchers at Dartmouth watched these reward-driven teen deci-sions unfold with brain scans. They presented adults and adolescents with scenarios like "setting your hair on fire," "jumping off a roof," and "swimming with sharks." Adults immediately assess those activities as not good ideas, whereas adolescents take longer to respond and use more limited brain regions in the process. Researchers refer to this as "gist" versus "verbatim" thinking. When faced with a scenario that could be

THE CASE FOR NOT BUBBLE WRAPPING

This drive for high rewards and low risk assessment might seem like an argument for bubble wrapping your child and protecting him until the forebrain fibers are connected. It's a tempting pros-pect, but now that we know more about adolescent curiosity, learning, and bravery, we can see it's better to channel, not limit, this wonderful drive. If we overly control our kids, they begin to lose their confidence and do not listen to their inner voice. People who feel no control over their lives can become depressed through a well-known psychological process called "learned helplessness," so even teens who are showered with every op-portunity and advantage can feel hopeless and sad if they do not feel in control or have a sense of agency. Risk-taking may make our hearts race as parents, but it's a strength that was preserved in human development because young people need to be able to explore their environment and grow.

Look for ways to give kids freedom to have adventures and put them in charge of their own lives and decisions, and more and more as time goes on they show greater capability (see chapter 7 for the Parent Fade and chapter 8 for ALP). Making mistakes is part of experimenting, developing a sense of self-determination, and learning something new. Our bravery and outside-the-box thinking in adolescence have allowed us to forge our own paths and to do things differently than what our parents did. From an evolutionary standpoint, this ability is part of what makes us uniquely human.

dangerous, adults tend to cut through the alluring distractions and get to the bottom line (the gist) and say, "No way!" They use intuition to make a judgment about whether something is a good idea. Adolescents are more likely to weigh and deliberate information in a more literal sense (the verbatim)—and focus heavily on the reward. Brain scans of adolescents also indicate that a region important in helping us detect our own mistakes—the anterior cingulate cortex—is not fully wired yet. This means that even if something goes wrong, it takes adolescents longer to learn from mistakes and monitor their own behavior. Connecting the dots takes more time and experience.

Poor sleep makes risky decisions more likely. When adolescents don't sleep enough, the collaboration between the upstairs and downstairs brain is reduced, which means rewards and impulse are even more influential than they naturally would be, because the oversight regions are offline. Not surprisingly, brain scans show that teens who sleep less take more risks, and while they are doing so, the prefrontal cortex is less active and areas involved in reward are more active.

SLEEP MAKES ADOLESCENTS EXPERTS

Anyone who has parented or taught a tween or teen has marveled at the speed with which they learn a new skill. Watching an adolescent quickly become an expert can be breathtaking. At age eleven, Heather's son picked up a skateboard—a challenge of balance, quick reaction, motor skill coordination, and courage. By the second day he was going full speed down the street (reluctantly wearing a massive amount of padding), and on the third day he was creating mini ramps in the yard. Trying to learn this new skill five years previously would have taken more time, and trying to learn this skill as an adult might end in frustration (and injury!).

How do adolescents learn so fast? It's partly because they have an

BRAIN DEVELOPMENT 101

What does it mean to say that the brain "remodels"? From babyhood through childhood and adolescence and into adulthood, there are many ways that the brain changes, including:

- Growing new brain cells (or neurons)
- Connecting brain cells to each other and creating pathways (or synapses)
- Letting unused pathways die off (pruning)
- Making well-used pathways faster and more efficient (myelination)

Growing new brain cells, or neurons, happens in utero. In fact, newborn babies have 100 billion brain cells—the densest brain they will ever have. When they come into the world, babies begin to form connections, or synapses, between neurons at an unimaginable pace of approximately a million synapses per second. These connections allow cells and regions of the brain to start to talk to each other and coordinate a baby's thoughts and movements. These synapses continue to form at a breathtaking speed and peak in early childhood.

At the same time, neurons and synapses die off, which is called pruning and helps make our brains the super processors that they are. Our brains are wide-open sponges of possibility, ready to learn and adapt. Human infants are able to launch into any environment, learn any language and set of behaviors and customs, with brains like ready-made laboratories. But their experiments start immediately, and as babies learn, they quickly become specialists in the world they have entered. The brain cells and connections that they use light up and strengthen, and the ones they don't use die off—which in turn funnels energy to the relevant and well-used cells and connections.

At first, the connections babies form are relatively slow (which is why an infant's reaction time is slower and their movements are uncoordinated and adorably clumsy). To make brain connections extraordinarily fast and efficient, a fatty layer develops around the connections—this is called "myelin," and it insulates the electrical impulses between brain cells and along pathways in the brain. Myelin allows strong and fast connections throughout the brain. A baby's brain stem (where basic functions like breathing, heartbeat, and sleep are controlled) is almost fully myelinated, but the rest of the brain is not.

In adolescence, the brain ramps up pruning, especially in the frontal lobes. It may sound like a bad thing, but pruning is what gives our brains their unique form and function. (As a ballpark guess for just how many connections are trimmed, the macaque monkey has been estimated to lose a whopping five thousand synapses per second in the preadult years.) Eventually, roughly half of the neurons and synapses are eliminated, largely in the frontal lobes. While pruning is in process, the myelin envelops the pathways and turns up the speed. Think of this like a town with many small, poky roads that over time lays down thoroughfares and highways connecting the most important and highly frequented places. This flashy, billion-dollar upgrade happens largely—that's right—while an adolescent is asleep.

In fact, sleep recordings of children's and adolescents' brains show this unique signature of pruning as the years progress. Pruning is thought to happen in deep sleep (NREM). As we will describe in chapter 3, the deeper sleep stages are more pronounced in later childhood and early adolescence, and then begin to slowly decline in power, starting with the lower regions of the brain and ending finally with the prefrontal cortex. This shows the decline in brain cells and connections—the result of pruning. Studies of ten- to thirty-year-olds measuring electrical activity in the brain through electroencephalograms (EEGs), as well as brain scans, show that during the second decade, the activity of the brain's gray matter (made up of brain cells) decreases significantly toward the front of the brain, ending in the mid-twenties.

Our brains form connections, prune, and myelinate throughout

(continued)

39

childhood, adolescence, and into young adulthood. The lower regions of the brain, where emotion, drive, and motivation are housed, are connected earlier in development. The prefrontal cortex—at the very front of the brain, right behind the forehead—is very slowly pruned and strengthened into a person's twenties or even thirties. This region is responsible for functions like perspective, judgment, self-control, planning, emotion regulation, and self-awareness. During adolescence, the frontal lobes and the prefrontal cortex continue to mature and strengthen their connections to the rest of the brain. This ultimately makes the brain a more integrated system and also gives the frontal lobes the ability to communicate better with the emotional areas of the brain.

Neural circuits in adolescence are primed and ready to learn, extremely plastic, reward seeking, and socially driven. This can be a wonderful advantage when it takes place against the backdrop of healthy sleep. As the frontal lobes mature and strengthen their connections to the rest of the brain, we can integrate all our new ideas and insights, and we get better at seeing the big picture. We become "wiser," learning from experience and making decisions based on a broader view. Protecting sleep during this turbulent time is essential.

abundance of *excitatory* connections (brain synapses that fire with a Go! signal) compared to *inhibitory* (Stop!) connections. Learning information and skills happens when brain cells "fire" together, and over time the connections between them become stronger, by way of a process called "long-term potentiation" (LTP). These excitatory connections and LTP make adolescents learning machines. Compared to children and adults, adolescents have the fastest reaction times. In lab studies, adolescents have superb memory performance (explaining why Heather can no longer beat her son at the game Memory). Another way to say this is that adolescents have high neural *plasticity*, meaning their brains are primed to change and grow.

During sleep, the brain takes the information it has learned during the day, sorts it, tags it, and processes it into long-term storage. Sleep deprivation interferes with learning in many ways, which we'll see clearly in chapter 5. Animal studies have shown that restricted sleep or fragmented sleep can reduce neurogenesis, or the growing and connecting of new brain cells. For example, kittens who have been allowed to see out of only one eye will regain their normal sight if they are allowed a lot of deep sleep.

This plasticity makes adolescence a prime time of life to practice and get good at things. How you spend your time really counts, as the brain circuits you use are strengthened, but the ones you don't are at risk of being pruned away. Improving your three-point shot, lowering your mile time, working on your fencing moves, or learning coding? Practice *and* good sleep are the winning combination.

Improving teenage sleep is essential to mental health, safety, and learning, yet every night, adolescents are missing out on the magical benefits of hours of this brain building, emotional balancing, and neural refinement. When you consider the psychological advantages and the implications for public health and safety—in the form of reduced stress, less potential violence, and fewer driving accidents, just to name a few—it's clear that the benefits of good sleep to teens, families, and society are enormous. Adopting healthy school schedules, promoting academic balance (both of which we will explore in chapter 5), and protecting teens' sleep at home (chapter 6) will fuel all these amazing brain powers and support adolescents so they can see the world as safe, fun, and full of hope and possibility.

3

Adolescent Sleep:
Understanding the Storm

Max was a thoughtful, active teen who simply could not sleep. As much as his parents tried to help him, he stayed up late—his mind racing and his body feeling so wound up it was impossible to relax. He tried listening to music, following the guided meditations his mom had suggested he install on his phone, and tracking his sleep with the watch his dad got him. Still, everyone else in the house would fall asleep and his mind would ramp up again. His parents worried that he had a real problem, and that his late-night pattern and lack of sleep were starting to affect his mood. During the school week, he woke up early every morning, and felt like he was in a fog. On the weekends, when he didn't have lacrosse practice, he could sleep until 11:00 a.m.

Summer came and Max went to sleepaway camp. Leaving his computer, phone, fitness tracker, and every other gadget he owned behind, he took off for the woods with his siblings. Within three nights, the formerly sleep-resistant night owl was falling asleep—deeply and peacefully—around 10:00 p.m., sleeping a long and restorative night, and waking easily with the group for a full day of activities. Why? You might assume it was the mental break from school and the hustle of everyday teenage life—and you'd be partially correct. The truth is, though, that the sleep correction Max experienced was as much biological as it was psychological. Max was experiencing what we call paleo-sleep—sleep in a natural setting, without technology, light, and all the other aspects of modern life—and his body's internal clock was reset. Almost without effort, his evolutionarily old sleep systems synced and breathed a sigh of relief. In this chapter we'll explore why and how this happened. Once you understand these natural sleep mechanisms, you'll see—even without a trip to summer camp—how you can harness these ideas and unleash the power of sleep.

THE RUMBLINGS OF AN APPROACHING STORM

Middle childhood is the sunny springtime of sleep. When kids are aged six to ten, the resistance to bedtime routines has often faded, nightmares are less frequent, and most school-age kids can go full speed all day long, running, swinging, reading, eating—and then naturally fall into a deep and long sleep. During this time, good sleep becomes the norm in many homes, and parents often forget it was ever a concern.

In adolescence, the pressure begins to build, and clouds of sleep loss move across the sky. This sweet honeymoon of sleep comes to an end.

In middle school, most kids lose their footing on healthy sleep habits. By age fifteen the vast majority are sleep deprived. A lab study of tenth graders showed that, when given the opportunity to sleep during the day, nearly half fell directly into REM sleep—a symptom normally associated with the sleep disorder narcolepsy. It took these kids an average of 3.4 minutes to fall asleep when given the chance at 8:30 a.m. (a time when the average high schooler might be expected to take a calculus test). One set of CDC data showed that 57 percent of middle schoolers in the U.S. do not meet the recommended number of hours of sleep, and in high school that rose to 93 percent.

Meanwhile, the severity of the problem goes largely unnoticed. Many parents don't realize how sleep deprived their teen is, and the nature of the mental and physical toll this takes on the body. Sleep is when growth hormone is secreted, muscles and tissues repair, and neural connections are refined and strengthened. Deep sleep sends soothing signals to the body's fight-or-flight system. Healthy sleep gives us an infusion of neuro-chemicals like dopamine (the reward chemical) and norepinephrine (akin to the brain's natural adrenaline), fueling us with positive energy. Our waking hours, on the other hand, are when stress hormones are higher and the body is taxed. When teens do not sleep enough, brain and body repair is cut short, positive neurochemicals are dampened, and the scales are tipped toward chronic stress. Regions of the brain, like the prefrontal cortex, that help us regulate emotions are dulled, which is why studies of even partially sleep-deprived people show they become more irritable, volatile, and negative.

Pioneering sleep researcher William Dement, known as the father of sleep medicine, once described sleep (or lack thereof) as creating our life's mood music. When you sleep well, the background music is upbeat and positive, so you interpret people's behaviors and daily events with humor and optimism. When you miss sleep, the mood music darkens, and suddenly people have questionable motives. Life takes on a more negative and gloomy tone.

As we saw in the previous chapter, research closely connects lost sleep with deteriorating mental health. A recent study of adolescents in the UK found that teens who slept less at age fifteen were significantly more likely to have symptoms of depression and anxiety at age seventeen and in their early twenties. Those diagnosed with depression went to bed later, woke up more during the night, and were more likely to say they felt very sleepy during the day than those without a mental health diagnosis. We are all discussing teen mental health, but sleep is a glaring hole in this conversation. To effectively address teen mental health is to address sleep. There's just no getting around it.

In the chapters that make up Part 1 of this book, we're exploring the reasons for such a drastic decline in teen sleep. This will lead us to the entry points for making changes and helping teenagers regain this vital component of their mental and physical health. It's important to understand that teens are sleep deprived because of multiple factors that converge and amplify one another during this phase of life. In this chapter, we'll look at the internal, biological factors. It turns out that adolescents have unique brain clocks, creating a rhythm that is different from that of younger kids and adults. This dictates a night owl tendency that legitimately and biologically delays the timing of their twenty-four-hour day. In chapters 4 and 5, we'll look at the external factors—omnipresent technology, early school start times, and academic overload—that swoop in and join forces with these internal biological ones. The crisis created by these internal and external factors is what eminent sleep researcher Mary Carskadon calls the "perfect storm." Regaining healthy teenage sleep means understanding how the storm is created.

THE DAZZLING POWERS OF TEENAGE SLEEP

Do you remember, as a teen, that you could stay awake into the wee hours and sleep deeply through the morning—sunlight streaming in the windows, neighborhood dogs barking, and other family members banging pots and pans in the kitchen? Many teens have zero interest in climbing into bed before midnight and can sleep through a fire drill in the early morning.

What's the reason for this teen nocturnal transformation? It's not rebellion or laziness—as we once might have thought. The answer starts with an interesting shift in the adolescent sleep clock—a neurological change that sets teenagers on a later rhythm than the rest of us.

What we know about the curious sleep patterns of adolescents began to unfold in the 1970s, with the work of Mary Carskadon and William Dement at Stanford University. To investigate how sleep changes through the preteen and adolescent years, the researchers created the Stanford Sleep Camp and embarked on a multiyear study. Starting with a group of ten-, eleven-, and twelve-year-olds, the researchers organized camp-like activities during the day and measured the kids' sleep at night. The same kids returned to campus in the summers for several years, giving a longitudinal view of how their sleep developed through adolescence.

What they expected was that kids would naturally sleep less as they got older. They were astounded to see this was not the case at all. At the beginning of the study, the preteens slept an average of 9.25 hours of the ten hours allotted. But every year they returned to sleep camp, they continued to sleep the same number of hours. Not only that, when they were younger, after nine or ten hours of sleep, the kids tended to wake up naturally and easily, and were alert when tested during the day. The older teenagers, on the other hand, despite also sleeping nine to ten hours, often had to be woken up in the morning (after an allotted ten-hour sleep period) and were less alert during the day. It was truly a surprise to see how much the older teens continued to sleep, and even with this long night of sleep, the data seemed to show they were drowsier than their younger counterparts.

Dr. Dement wrote that one of his first takeaways from the early years of the sleep camp was just how alert and well rested the preteens were. He described them as "like puppies, bursting with energy; at night they slept about 10 hours," and referred to this age as the pinnacle of sleep perfection. Seeing that the older adolescents, by measures taken in the lab, were sleepier during the day initially led Carskadon and Dement to think that teens might need about an hour more sleep than younger kids. They later revised their thinking to reflect that the drowsiness resulted from the sleep debt these older teens carried (even though they were instructed to sleep for ten hours a night the week before the lab assessments), as well as the developmental force we'll explore in a moment—the natural timing shift in the teen sleep clock.

Regardless, the adolescents averaged about nine and a quarter hours at every age. Since these classic studies, much more research has backed up this need for an average of nine to ten hours per night through adolescence.

This remarkable desire for sleep has amazed scientists and parents alike. In lab studies, researchers have seen just how long teens' bodies want to sleep, if given the chance. In a later study, Carskadon found that teenagers, studied in the lab for three nights, given an eighteen-hour opportunity to sleep, slept an average of nearly 12.5 hours the first night (again, a sign of teens making up for lack of sleep) and 10.1 hours by the third night. Most parents tell us they too are in awe of their teen's sleeping powers. A dad joked recently that over the summer, his two teenage boys were like cats—coming out to eat and then disappearing again, back to bed. On holidays, Heather has seen her young adolescent routinely sleep eleven hours and still need a nudge to get out of bed. In fact, as a young adult, Julie's son can still sleep ten hours at night. If they're allowed to sleep to their body's full desire, many kids will sleep even more at age sixteen than they did at age ten.

If this sounds surprising, consider how much sense it makes. As we have learned, the brain and body are going through massive transformations during adolescence, and much of this transformation in the brain happens during sleep. Remember when you worked so hard to get your baby sleeping on a schedule, or you noticed your toddler became hyper and overtired, so you created an elaborate bedtime routine to help him wind down? We take such good care of our little ones' sleep because we know their brains are exploding with growth. Teenagehood is the same. Changes related to puberty and a reorganization of the brain mean that the period of adolescence, similar to earlier massive developmental explosions, is a time when sleep becomes *more* important, not less. Meanwhile, recent estimates put the average teen at a loss of about two hours of sleep every school night.

SLEEP ON THE DECLINE

A study of middle and high schoolers in the 1990s found their average sleep time was 7.53 hours, which is less than optimal sleep, but nearing adequate levels. By 2006, that number had dwindled by half an hour. An analysis of 270,000 middle and high schoolers found that between 1996 and 2012, there was a significant rise in the percentage of kids who slept less than seven hours per night, and the greatest drop-off in sleep time was in the fifteen-year-olds. By grade 12, the average kid sleeps about 6.5 hours on school nights. A survey from 2020, during the pandemic, put the high school senior year average at 6.4 hours.

This decline in sleep seems to be occurring at all ages, though. Data suggests children in general sleep an hour and a half less than they did in the twentieth century. In the 1940s, Gallup poll data showed the average American adult slept just shy of eight hours per night. Now it's 6.8. Sleep researcher Robert Stickgold once told *Harvard Magazine*: "We are living in the middle of history's greatest experiment in sleep deprivation and we are all a part of that experiment."

DECODING THE ADOLESCENT SLEEP CLOCK

Now we understand the remarkable abilities teens have to sleep when given the chance. But despite this huge biological thirst for sleep, teens do tend to naturally stay up later than their younger siblings and often their parents. The average bedtime as kids move through middle and high school goes from 9:00 p.m. to 11:00 p.m. or midnight, and some stay up much later than that. A mom of four recently told us that on weekends and school breaks, her oldest teen goes into "vampire mode" and sleeps from 3:00 a.m. to 3:00 p.m. During the pandemic, we heard anecdotes of teens staying up until all hours of the morning and then signing into their online school just a few hours later, still in bed and half-asleep.

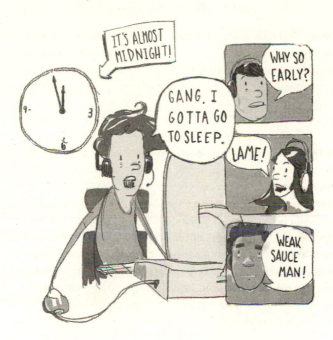

CIRCADIAN RHYTHMS AND THE "SLEEP PHASE DELAY": THE TEEN BRAIN MARCHING TO ITS OWN BEAT

This late-night tendency is due to a shift in the teen sleep clock. To understand this change and how it affects our teens, let's look at how sleep is generated in the first place. For all humans, sleep is controlled by two processes: the circadian rhythms and the homeostatic sleep drive. It's important to understand these two processes, because they both change in adolescence.

The **circadian rhythms** are the biological timekeeper in the body. They have a genetic and chemical system that keeps time, just like a clock that continues to tick on its own to let us know what time of day it is. The circadian rhythms are made by a pair of neuron clusters called the "suprachiasmatic nuclei" (SCN), located in the hypothalamus region of the brain. These clusters of brain cells perform as the "master clock"—a timekeeper that generates a twenty-four-hour cycle. The SCN sends signals to all other cells and organs throughout the body to coordinate the timing of our systems. Heart cells have clocks, liver cells have clocks, and so on. The master clock synchronizes the multiple clocks in other tissues throughout the body. Clocks in the digestive system know that we eat around a certain time, so our tummy begins to grumble, and clocks in our neurological system know when we'll need energy and when we'll need to wind down. These clocks affect when we are tired, alert, creative, and hungry, as well as our body temperature, metabolism, and other physiological processes.

When the brain's clock knows that night is coming, the hormone melatonin is released, signaling the time for sleep is approaching, allowing us to wind down, become drowsy, and let sleep take over. Toward biological morning, the brain sends signals to tell us, "It's day!" Melatonin levels go down and cortisol and other activating hormones rise. We become alert, productive, and ready to enjoy the day.

Little kids' circadian rhythms, otherwise known as their internal clocks, tell them to go to bed early and wake up early. Most little kids can fall asleep at 8:00 p.m. and be awake and ready to play around 6:00 a.m. As kids enter adolescence, though, they experience a natural shift to a later biological timing. This is not just a preference; it happens at a chemical level. Studies measuring the melatonin levels of adolescents have found that these rise about two hours later than younger kids' (pushing natural bedtime and natural wake time two hours later as well). This phenomenon of shifting to a later rhythm is called a "sleep phase delay." The sleep phase delay has been linked to the onset of puberty, suggesting that something in the neurological and chemical changes related to puberty

WHAT PARENTS TELL US
ABOUT THE TEEN SLEEP CLOCK

It takes Emerson longer to fall asleep and I usually have to drag him out of deep sleep in the morning. I've noticed he is needing more sleep lately. Growing all those mustache hairs takes it out of you, I guess.

Ava will stay asleep unless Harry Styles is dropping a new video, she has school/practice, or we wake her up.

Cooper could sleep all day if I didn't wake him up at 7:30. After that, he's still a walking, grunting zombie.

Over the summer, Raiss started going to bed really late, like midnight or later. Then he'd wake up around noon or 1 p.m. We couldn't change his sleep pattern to save our lives. Now that he's back to school, he falls asleep around eleven, and then we have to set a bomb off in his room to wake him in the morning.

triggers the delay in the master clock. The brain becomes paced differently, and from a chemical standpoint, the biological night of an adolescent is shifted later. This is key to understanding how to support teenagers' sleep: the brain tells them to go to bed later and wake up later than young kids and grown-ups. From a chemical standpoint (and given all that is on their plate), most are unable to fall asleep early enough to regularly get eight to ten hours of nightly sleep. High schools that start at 7:45 a.m. or even 8:00 a.m. go hand in hand with sleep deprivation.

This sleep phase delay means that an eight-year-old might be drowsy and ready to sleep by 8:00 p.m., but an adolescent is physically unable to fall asleep for the night until about 10:00 p.m. or later. This delayed timing also means that teens are not physiologically ready to wake up until later than the eight-year-old. As all parents know, little kids are prone to early rising, ready to build Legos and do cartwheels at 6:00 a.m. or earlier. In

CIRCADIAN RHYTHMS

Since the birth of our planet, the sun has been rising and setting daily, and nearly all forms of life have adapted rhythms to these day and night patterns. These circadian (from the Latin *circa*, meaning "around," and *diem*, meaning "day") rhythms help living beings coordinate the timing of all their intricate biological systems and anticipate what will be needed at different times of the day. Honeybees use their internal clocks to time their visits to flowers. Flowers themselves use internal clocks to "remember" when to open petals and even when to release the most potent smells.

In humans, the internal clock is reliable, but it's not precisely set to twenty-four hours. The average adolescent and adult internal day length has been measured at 24.2 hours. This means that, without signals from the sun, the internal clock would run on a slightly longer cycle. Left to its own devices, a teen's internal clock would be out of sync with reality in no time, turning day into night and night into day. Thankfully, the sun, along with signals like eating breakfast, chatting with family, experiencing darkness, and changes in temperature, keep the internal clock on track. These constant reminders and corrections to the clock are called "entrainment"—the factors from the outside world keeping the internal clock in sync. If it sounds weird or inconvenient that our internal clock needs constant reminders, it's actually a good thing. It means that we are able to adjust our internal clocks as the timing of sunrise and sunset and the length of the night change with the seasons. This is also why, after a number of days, we can adapt to other time zones after travel.

However, as modern humans, we abuse this built-in adaptability. Our circadian rhythms are no longer being nudged gently as the seasons change. Instead we blow them out of the water with powerful signals of light and activity at unnatural times. These forces upend our finely tuned natural system. We can easily fool our internal clocks and stay up late—with bright home lights, computers, social media, and video games. In fact, this late-night light and activity can actually give us a spike in stress hormones. When we stay up late, our brain naively tries to help us, perhaps because it thinks we must be in danger (why else would we be awake in the middle of the night?). This kicks off more anxiety and adrenaline, which keep us awake and can cause insomnia.

In general, as modern humans, we don't have anywhere near as much sunlight during the day as the human brain evolved with, nor do we have anywhere near as much darkness at night. It's easy to see how the brain—which controls our sleep—can become confused. This is why our troubled teen, Max, was alert and wired when he wanted to be sleeping, but when he went to camp, the sun and darkness allowed him to sync up his natural sleep systems.

Our brain has an alerting function called the "reticular activating system" nestled deep in the brain stem, with projections all over the various regions of the brain. When we sleep enough and have a regular schedule, the activating system triggers neurochemicals like dopamine to infuse the brain with positive energy and motivation. When this activating system falters or is dampened by too little sleep or a confused circadian clock, the effect is lower desire and motivation—less zest for life.

Circadian rhythms are so integral to our health that in 2017, three scientists won the Nobel Prize in Physiology or Medicine for their discoveries of molecular mechanisms controlling the circadian rhythms.

fact, the younger the child, the earlier they tend to start the day. But as kids reach adolescence, what was once gymnastics hour is now still the biological night. In fact, as we will see later in this chapter, the early-morning hours for adolescents contain intense and valuable stages of sleep, including dreams—making this important sleep time. This explains why a fire engine could drive through the bedroom and a teen could keep sleeping peacefully: 6:00 a.m. is still the night, according to a teenager's sleep clock.

Our preference for morning or evening is called our "chronotype," or you might hear people describe it as being an early bird or night owl.

Most adolescents shift into evening chronotypes, or night owls, in a clear way. Parents of these teens and the teens themselves tell us it's very hard to imagine falling asleep before 11:00 p.m. and it's very hard to wake up in the morning. A smaller subset seems to keep a morning tendency—such as our friend's sixteen-year-old who can fall asleep at 10:00 p.m. and wake early and easily for school. These teens tend to grow into adults who likewise prefer early schedules. For most teens, the evening preference begins around age twelve and reaches its peak for girls at age 19.5, and for boys at age twenty-one. In our twenties, we tip back toward a morning preference again. This is a phenomenon that has been observed across cultures around the world. In fact, researchers have also measured a sleep phase delay in other mammals that coincides with sexual maturation, which backs up the biological nature of the teen sleep delay. Rhesus monkeys, marmosets, and mice, for example, experience a delay in their internal clock around the time of puberty.

How the Modern Environment Is Conspiring Against Teen Sleep

So then, gaming and video chatting with friends past midnight is just natural? Should we let teens do this if it's what their brain clock dictates? Not so fast. The sleep phase delay *naturally* shifts teenagers' sleep somewhat later, but light, technology, school, and social forces prey on this natural delay, adding an additional delay and pushing sleep times to an *unnatural* and often unhealthy point. The environment takes advantage of and accentuates the sleep phase delay and keeps teenagers awake way beyond a natural bedtime. To allow our paleo-sleep to emerge, we have to put down the VR headset and step away from the phone. (As we'll discuss in chapter 6, it's important to do this about an hour before bed to allow the prelude to sleep.) Generally speaking, light exposure in the evening will convince the brain it's still day and will delay drowsiness.

Light suppresses the release of sleep-inducing chemicals like melatonin. Remember, over hundreds of thousands of years, our eyes and brains evolved to respond to sunlight as an indicator that it's daytime and we should be alert, but now computer screens, phones, and even interior home lights can send the same signals. All these sources of light, along with the mental stimulation of social media, games, video chats with friends, and so forth can increase arousal and suppress sleep chemistry. (We will look specifically at screens and sleep in chapter 4.)

To make matters worse, research has pointed to adolescents being more sensitive to evening light and therefore prone to an accentuated delay in falling asleep. Younger adolescents ages eleven to fourteen have been shown to be incredibly sensitive to evening light. In fact, the melatonin of young adolescents was shown to be suppressed to a surprising degree even with relatively low levels of light in the evening. This means the young adolescent circadian rhythms may be particularly easy to trick—with bright iPad screens and engrossing games. When this happens, kids legitimately don't feel tired, and if they climb into bed, they might lie there awake, tossing and turning. To a large degree, this explains why teen sleep has declined alarmingly in recent years, as we have ever more sources of light and diversion from our homes and devices.

On the other hand, sunlight in the morning causes an "advance" and sets the circadian rhythms earlier, putting us on an earlier schedule and making us sleepy earlier in the evening. These "delaying" and "advancing" effects are a really important takeaway for adolescents and parents. Teenagers need less light in the evening and more light (sunlight is the absolute best) in the morning, to keep their brain clocks in sync. Otherwise the sleep phase delay becomes a runaway train. Morning sunlight keeps the train on the tracks, constantly nudging and sending alerting "go" signals to internal clocks to keep them more in sync with the schedules imposed by school, and to somewhat counteract the tendency to become delayed. It's amazing that morning sunlight starts a timer in the brain that sets the stage for the sleep that will come fifteen or so hours later; but it's true, morning sun makes it easier to fall asleep at bedtime. The cells in our eyes that set the circadian rhythms respond best to the sun, so turning on the lights in your house does not have as strong an effect. When your teen wakes, she should spend a short amount of time outside. In sunny climates, five to ten minutes of outdoor sun in the morning may suffice. In other areas, more time may be needed to have the same effect, although the sun through clouds is still stronger than interior home lights. This is challenging on short days in the wintertime, which may result in darkness into the waking day, especially if school starts early—and even more so at higher latitudes. In this case, later school start times, starting the school day with outside time (see page 59), and a light source designed to mimic sunlight, may be needed.

A good rule of thumb for teens is to go outside for breakfast, walk to school if possible, spend first period outside (hint to schools), and sit outside or go for a walk or a run before 10:00 a.m. on the weekends. After morning has passed, the circadian rhythms have moved on and light will no longer advance the clock. If a teen's normal wake-up time is 7:00 a.m., then the internal clock will respond to morning sun for a couple of hours after this, but going outside at noon is unlikely to help. In the evening, lowering the lights in the home, turning off computers, and putting away phones is key to allowing a natural rise in melatonin, which invites the body to fall asleep easily.

Camping Studies Show Us Our Natural Sleep Potential

Imagine our ancestors, who rose with the sun and the sounds of birdcalls and spent their days hunting and foraging, feeling naturally sleepy after darkness fell and the temperature dropped. We evolved, at a cellular level, to take our cues from the bright sun and the dark nights, and from the slowly changing seasonal patterns. And while we still operate with the same biological systems as our ancestors, we no longer have the natural cues that helped them sleep: we're inside most of the day in artificial lights, which are very different in intensity, color, and angle than the sun, and often these lights stay on during what should be night. The exquisitely timed rhythms of the day and night are confused by all these modern signals.

Researcher Kenneth Wright, at the University of Colorado Boulder, has studied how the body responds when it returns to nature, by conducting a series of camping experiments. In one, participants spent a summer weekend without the use of lamps or flashlights and without personal electronic devices, minus any source of light except the natural sun, starlight, moonlight, and campfires. After this short trip in nature, when the campers returned, their saliva was tested, and melatonin was rising 1.4 hours earlier than before they left. In another experiment, campers went out for a week during the winter solstice—the longest night of the year—while a control group stayed home. During the six days in nature, they also experienced the long night without artificial light. The campers' melatonin shifted earlier by 2.6 hours—lining up more closely with natural sunset. During the day, these winter campers got thirteen times more light than the control group (who were home in mostly artificial light), and at night they slept an average of almost ten hours per night, or 2.3 hours more than their counterparts who were at home. Fascinatingly, both summer and winter campers slept more or less in line with sunset and sunrise—suggesting that humans adapt to seasonal sleep patterns as the length of day and the temperature changes. Circadian biologist Horacio de la Iglesia and researchers at the University of Washington saw this when they measured the sleep of two historically hunter-gatherer indigenous communities in Argentina—one with access to electricity and one without. Those in the community with electricity slept less than those who had only natural light, but in both communities, sleep time was longer in the winter than in the summer. This seasonal adaptability has been seen in other species: hamsters and sheep have a longer period of high melatonin levels in the winter versus the summer. It's likely that humans also have this natural mechanism for taking in more sleep during darker, cooler winter months, but because of our modern lifestyles and artificial lighting, we're not in touch with this adaptability.

THE SLEEP DRIVE: WHY YOUR TEEN GETS A SECOND WIND AFTER YOU'VE GONE TO BED

Going back to our two basic sleep processes, the second is the **homeostatic sleep drive**. The concept of the sleep drive is simple: the longer we are awake, the greater the pressure to sleep. Throughout the day, the pressure to sleep continues to build until our bedtime, when the pressure is greatest. This pressure is related to the buildup of a chemical called adenosine, which is a by-product of burning energy (ATP). By the end of the day (or sooner, if we're sleep deprived), high concentrations of adenosine make sleep irresistible. While we sleep, adenosine is cleared and the pressure dissipates slowly until morning. If our sleep drive was acting alone, we would get progressively more tired as the day went on, until the pressure to sleep would be overwhelming, but this doesn't happen thanks to our circadian rhythms, which sends us alerting signals late in the day to give us a last burst of energy and help us stay awake in the evening. This is why we often feel drowsy in the midafternoon but get a second wind before dinnertime and are able to stay awake until bedtime. The late-day alerting signals of the internal clock are withdrawn before bedtime so that the sleep pressure can take over and we can get a full night's sleep. When the sleep drive and the circadian rhythms are aligned, people sleep well. When they are misaligned, both sleep and alertness are compromised.

We know that the teen circadian rhythms are delayed, but a remarkable change in the homeostatic sleep pressure system also happens in adolescence: sleep pressure builds up more slowly across the day, which makes it easier for teens to stay awake longer than the rest of us. For toddlers, the sleep pressure builds up so fast that a nap is needed, and a young child who has stayed up all day will crash at an early bedtime. This is not the case for teens. The slower buildup of sleep pressure, accompanied by the sleep phase delay, means that a teen's second wind might start to ramp up at 9:00 p.m.—giving a burst of alertness, the desire to stay awake, the ability to study, or new energy to engage with friends or technology. At this point, sleep is a distant dream.

Already, we can see how multiple internal forces conspire to make teens go to bed later: a natural delay in the internal clock, along with a sensitivity to evening light and a slower buildup of sleep pressure. From here, it's easy to see why the external world and the habits of modern teen life create the perfect storm and push sleep to an unhealthy point.

Commonly, teens tell us they just cannot fall asleep at a good hour. This often has to do with social jet lag (which we'll discuss shortly), but it's also because it's extremely hard for a teenager to wind down and fall asleep, given the forces of biology and the stimulation from school responsibilities, social life, work, lights, technology, and more. It's tempting to let teens get swept up in this storm, but given the negative consequences of poor sleep, this should instead be a wake-up call to take extra precautions to manage evening light and screens and excessive homework (which is also often on screens), set school start times later, estab-

PRACTICAL TAKEAWAY FOR SLEEP-FORWARD SCHOOLS

The natural bright light of the sun is in large part what keeps our circadian clocks happy and in sync. Classrooms should have as much sunlight as possible, and changes to schedules can include morning sunlight to allow the forces of nature to help kids stay alert and regulate their internal clocks. Students should start the day outside, in physical education or otherwise, to press go on the internal clock, and have many breaks or class activities outside when possible. Eat breakfast at the lunch tables outside, or have class discussions or writing exercises outside, especially in the first half of the day, whenever possible. This will help them be alert in class and also fall asleep easier at night. When kids go straight into a building with no sunlight in the morning, they do not get these helpful biological signals and their internal clocks remain out of sync.

PRACTICAL TAKEAWAY FOR SLEEP-FORWARD LEGISLATORS: PERMANENT *STANDARD* TIME

Currently, Congress is considering a bill to move the country to permanent daylight saving time. It does make sense to eliminate the time change and the negative health effects that come with shifting times twice every year. Humans are built to adapt slowly with the gradually changing seasons, not to make a sudden artificial clock shift.

However, scientists have made it clear that we should shift to permanent *standard* time, not permanent daylight saving time. Standard time (which is "normal" time) is a more natural rhythm, and is more in line with circadian biology. For adolescents this is a particularly important issue. The artificial delay of DST means very long, dark mornings, which is unhealthy, as the brain and body do not experience sun in the morning. In Seattle, for example, circadian biologists note this could be devastating for a depressed teenager in the winter.

---

lish an earlier and regular bedtime, and help teens start the day outside. More of these healthy sleep habits for families and schools can be found in chapters 4, 5, and 6.

SOCIAL JET LAG: A TUG OF WAR IN AN ADOLESCENT'S BODY

The teen sleep clock is biologically set later, but middle and high schools have not gotten the memo (or as we'll see in chapter 5, they might have gotten it, but tucked the memo away in a file cabinet). In an ironic twist, many high schools start earlier than elementary schools. This poses a terrible problem for an adolescent's brain and leads to a huge pileup of weekly sleep debt. It also leads to the social jet lag. Social jet lag refers to the discrepancy between the circadian clock and the social clock. On school days, wake-up times, classes, exams, and meals take place at odd times for the internal clock (*Why are you eating breakfast, it's still night-time! Why are you asking me to solve a math problem, I should be in REM sleep!*). This is like when we fly to another time zone and for a few days feel hungry, tired, or wired at the wrong times, and have a general feeling of being out of sorts. All the physiological processes that are controlled by the internal clock—the timing of hormones; the functioning of the heart, liver, and other organs—have trouble synchronizing and create a stress response that makes us feel bad.

On the weekends, many teens return to what is likely a more natural, later timing for their bodies, and they also attempt to make up for sleep that was lost during the week. If a teen sleeps seven hours a night during the week but she needs nine, this leads to an accumulation of ten hours

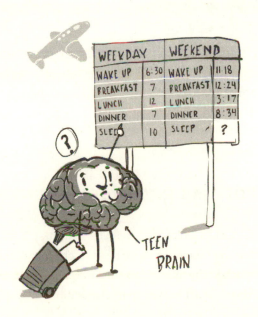

WEEKDAY		WEEKEND	
WAKE UP	6:30	WAKE UP	11:18
BREAKFAST	7	BREAKFAST	12:24
LUNCH	12	LUNCH	3:17
DINNER	7	DINNER	8:34
SLEEP	10	SLEEP	?

TEEN BRAIN

of sleep debt by the end of the school week. Understandably, on the weekends, she listens to her body's clock and sleeps later and longer—making up an average of two hours of sleep each weekend morning (and carrying over an average of six hours to the next week), but this makes it extra hard to fall asleep on Sunday night. Monday morning comes, and it's hard to feel alert. The internal clock is yet again confused and struggles to readjust. It's as if our kids fly cross-country twice a week, with their biology continually taxed as it tries to keep up with the jet lag. As we'll look at more closely in chapter 5, early school start times are the main culprit in social jet lag. In fact, research shows that moving start times even by one hour reduces social jet lag and increases student health and well-being.

SYMPTOMS OF SOCIAL JET LAG

- Daytime fatigue
- Weight gain (over time)
- Difficulty concentrating/functioning
- Digestive problems
- Mood changes
- General sense of not being well
- Chronic health conditions
- And ironically—insomnia

We can't entirely make up for lost sleep—it's not like a bank account we can just transfer money into later when we finally get it. The wear and tear on the body still happens during periods of sleep deprivation, and we can't necessarily reverse that process. But we can experience "rebound sleep"—sleeping deeper and more after a night of poor-quality sleep—so the body does have mechanisms for taking in more sleep when it's missing. It does feel magical to finally get a good night's sleep. Overall, though, the idea of catch-up sleep doesn't work very well, because of social jet lag.

Jet lag causes an asynchrony in the body and has serious consequences. Large-scale epidemiological studies have shown that social jet lag is linked to an increased body mass index (BMI) and that it raises the risk for many chronic diseases, including diabetes and heart problems. Psychological disorders like depression and bipolar disorder have been connected to disrupted daily rhythms as well. Animal studies have shown the effects of this clock disruption. For example, when rats are forced into a schedule that is out of sync with their master clock (for instance, a twenty-two- instead of a twenty-four-hour day), they exhibit classic signs of depression. Mice kept in twenty- versus twenty-four-hour day cycles gain excessive weight, and show hormonal disruptions and a loss of neurons in the prefrontal cortex of the brain.

Human beings of all ages thrive on regularity because our brains and bodies are always coordinating a complex orchestra of cells, tissues, or-

OPTIMAL VERSUS ADEQUATE SLEEP

Data from the Youth Risk Behavior Survey has consistently found that teens who don't sleep at least eight hours per night are at higher risk for using cigarettes, marijuana, or alcohol; being sexually active; seriously considering suicide; feeling sad or hopeless; physically fighting; being more sedentary; drinking more soda; and having more screen time. ADD symptoms also increase with poor sleep. Quite an exhaustive list of parental concerns, big and small—but this is the power of sleep.

Just as with adults, adolescents have varying sleep needs—some need slightly less, some slightly more. The need for sleep may also ebb and flow during adolescence. Research and clinical experience suggest that for most teens, nine to ten hours per night is "optimal," and eight to 8.5 hours per night may be "adequate."

gans, and systems. Imagine an orchestra conductor trying to do her job, but the string section is late, the horns leave early, and the percussion strikes up just at the end. The music would sound more like a cacophony than a symphony. Likewise, the body's genes and chemistry are all trying to work in harmony, but they rely on regular waking, light, eating, exercise, social time, and sleep to do so.

Even a few days of sleep deprivation or circadian misalignment in young, healthy volunteers increases appetite and caloric intake, levels of inflammatory markers, blood pressure, and evening cortisol levels, as well as insulin and blood glucose.

TEENAGERS MISSING THEIR DREAMS

Underslept teens accumulate ten or more hours of missing brain construction every week. Exactly how this is affecting their health and well-being is not fully understood, but it's likely we're seeing just the tip of the iceberg. The truncated sleep teens experience as they stay up late, wake early for school, and weather social jet lag accompany many of the changes in behavior we see as issues with teens: moodiness, apathy, negative thoughts and feelings, or conflicts and family disharmony. This is not a coincidence.

Let's imagine a teen is allowed glorious, optimal sleep: most would sleep around nine hours, beginning at roughly 10:00 or 11:00 p.m. Through the course of a full night, growth hormone is secreted and the body repairs, grows, and strengthens. The brain sifts through, transfers, and stores memories; clears toxins; repairs muscles; balances emotions; and more. After a full night's sleep, all of the dynamic work of sleep is complete and kids start the day with a full tank, ready to learn and take on challenges, and seeing the world through positive eyes. Here, our kids are like a group of Stanford University swimmers who extended their sleep time to ten hours in bed. They felt boosted mood, had more energy and faster reaction times, and also shaved time off their sprints (and if you watch the summer Olympics, you know a fraction of a second matters).

So what happens when the alarm goes off two hours before a teen is ready to wake up? For that answer, we can look at how sleep naturally unfolds through the night. In the beginning of the night, our sleep is predominantly non-REM (NREM), or deep sleep. As the night goes on, the proportion of NREM decreases and our REM sleep, or dream sleep, increases. In the early morning, we have less deep sleep, and our sleep time becomes dominated by dreams. (See more about "sleep architecture" on page 66.)

If adolescents sleep from 12:00 p.m. to 6:30 a.m., they miss roughly one-quarter of their total night's sleep. But this amputated morning sleep means they miss around half of their REM sleep, because the morning hours are the ones normally rich in dream sleep.

The consequences of routinely missing REM sleep are not fully understood, but we have every reason to think this is especially harmful to a teen's learning and mental health. Perhaps because of how random and unconstrained our associations are during REM, this stage of sleep helps us with our creativity, enabling us to understand complex problems and come up with new solutions. Dream sleep is vital to emotional health. During REM, emotional and memory centers of the brain, like the amygdala and hippocampus, are active, and the action of dream sleep seems to be in part to review and process our daytime experiences. Far from being entertainment or downtime for the brain, dream sleep helps us sort through and deal with the events in our lives. Researchers have shown that, when deprived of REM sleep, people start to lose their emotional compass—becoming less accurate at recognizing facial expressions and decoding what others are feeling. Without REM, they are more likely to perceive threats and are skewed toward fear-based reactions. If we want adolescents to feel hopeful and positive, we should take seriously the hours of emotional processing they lose every morning when

STAGES OF SLEEP: SLEEP ARCHITECTURE

In a sense, being asleep is just as active a state as being awake. Each stage of sleep plays a unique and vital role in promoting different aspects of growth and physical and mental health. The basic structure of sleep is called "sleep architecture." Dramatic changes in brain waves and chemistry distinguish the different sleep stages from one another and make up this architecture.

Humans cycle through all the stages of sleep approximately every ninety minutes throughout the night (the cycle is closer to sixty minutes for babies), including:

NREM (NON-RAPID EYE MOVEMENT)

During sleep, our temperature drops, muscles relax, and breathing and heart rate slow. NREM sleep starts out the night, descending from light to deep sleep. In NREM, brain waves are more regular and synchronized. During NREM sleep, memories and information are transferred from short-term to long-term storage, so this slow-wave sleep helps consolidate memories. It's harder to wake up a person in deep sleep. This stage of sleep is important for the process of "pruning" or getting rid of unused connections in the brain to divert space and energy to the important and used connections. In deep sleep, growth hormone is secreted. Growth hormones help cells divide and build and repair tissues. During childhood and adolescence, there is an increase in the nighttime secretion of growth hormone. In the deepest stages of sleep, the immune system is boosted.

"Sleep spindles" are an intriguing phenomenon that occur during NREM sleep. Sleep spindles are sudden bursts of brain waves that occur against the backdrop of regular NREM brain activity. There is exciting new evidence indicating that sleep spindles play a key role in memory formation and cognitive functioning. Adolescents exhibit a sharp increase in the frequency of sleep spindles. Data from multiple studies shows a relationship between higher spindle activity and intelligence, memory, and executive function. Like so many aspects of sleep, the exact function of sleep spindles is a topic of intriguing research—but it's likely that the intensity of spindles in the teen years is related to the magnitude of learning during this time. The last two hours of sleep are spindle rich (yes, the same two hours many teens are missing). In another interesting plot twist, sleep spindles play a role in protecting us from waking due to noise. We adults have fewer sleep spindles than teens, which could be why we pop awake when a floorboard creaks but teens need a foghorn to wake them up.

REM (RAPID EYE MOVEMENT)

In REM sleep, we have fast and erratic brain waves similar to awake brain waves. REM sleep is when we dream. Our eyes go back and forth under our lids—giving rapid eye movement sleep its name. REM sleep plays a role in strengthening the connections in the brain that are being used during the day—meaning that REM is also important for learning. In REM, our thoughts, feelings, experiences, images, and memories are all activated in random, bizarre orders, as if the brain is replaying an abstract show of our days. One take on dreams is that they are an important way that humans process emotions, integrate experiences, solidify information, and generally make sense of life. Dream sleep is also thought to feed our creativity and help us put ideas together in new ways. Thankfully, during REM sleep, our voluntary muscles are inactive (so we do not act out dreams), except in the case of certain sleep disorders.

Babies spend half their sleep time in REM sleep, and this turns out to be important for the formation of new brain connections. The proportion of NREM to REM sleep shifts from 50/50 in infancy, to 70/30 in childhood and 80/20 in adolescence.

they are forced out of bed too early. Many teens can easily fall asleep in the morning (anyone who has driven car pool knows this), and in the lab, measurements show that many will fall into REM sleep, as happens in narcolepsy, a sleep disorder. This is a teen's brain trying to pull them back into the dream sleep they are missing.

DEEP SLEEP, GROWTH, AND REMODELING

Deep sleep is also of vital importance. During deep sleep, growth hormone is secreted into the bloodstream. Growth hormone stimulates cell division and protein synthesis and helps to supply energy for tissue repair. The building and repairing of muscles and other tissues in the body is impossible without deep sleep. Growth hormone surges during adolescent sleep. The chemical that triggers the release of growth hormone also promotes sleep—so sleeping and growing go hand in hand. With all the growing they have to do, it's no surprise that teens need so much sleep.

As we saw in chapter 2, the frontal lobes of the brain—where judgment, insight, and other sophisticated brain functions are housed—prune, strengthen, and integrate with the rest of the brain during adolescence. And much of this brain development happens while a teen is asleep. In fact, changes in an adolescent's brain are often signaled by a few weeks of altered deep sleep intensity. This relationship has fascinating and powerful implications. It means sleep isn't just restoring, it appears to be *causing* development. Abnormalities in teens' deep sleep waves have been connected to faulty pruning (the process of removing connections gone wrong) in the frontal lobes, which is seen in psychiatric disorders like schizophrenia. Sleep studies have shown that the deep sleep waves of NREM seem to prune and integrate the back of the brain first. Over the years, the remodeling action of deep sleep moves toward the front of the brain. This lines up with what we know about how childhood brain powers transform in adolescence, with the frontal regions of the brain becoming more strongly connected and efficient, and the brain's powers of reasoning and judgment being some of the last to mature. It takes years of deep sleep for these sophisticated thinking skills to unfold to their highest potential.

As the brain's prefrontal regions strengthen and integrate with the rest of the brain, this continues to create wisdom and emotional balance in the adolescent years. But those abilities may not have the chance to develop properly under chronic sleep deprivation. This can make adolescents more vulnerable to mental health issues.

Deep sleep is also important in solidifying memories, which is why studies have shown that after a nap, or a night's sleep, people are better able to remember information. This is why it's better to go to bed than pull an all-nighter before a test.

So what stages or type of sleep are most important to adolescents? Sorry to break the news, but all of them. Deep sleep for memory, growth, and repair; sleep spindles for information transfer and learning; dream sleep for creativity and mental health (and the list could go on). There is no way to skimp on sleep without losing out on these benefits.

Now that we understand the basics of sleep and the internal, biological factors that make the teen sleep clock tick, we will see how these factors are swept up in the winds of the outside world to create a sleep-stealing storm. In the next chapter, we'll see how screens and technology take advantage of the adolescent night owl biology, and in the following chapter, how schools have become a major source of pressure squeezing a teenager's sleep from both sides. These explorations will help us see how teens and parents can take control of and improve their own sleep, and how teachers, school principals, and policy makers can make changes to support them.

TROUBLESHOOTING PARENTS' COMMON QUESTIONS ABOUT TEEN SLEEP

My teenager says if he gets into bed at the right time, he just lies there and can't fall asleep.

This is a really common dilemma for adolescents, and it's likely that your teen is right—he legitimately doesn't have the right sleepy chemicals on his side in order to fall asleep. Very often the cause of difficulty falling asleep is a case of social jet lag (meaning the internal clock is out of sync with school schedules, or confused by moving bedtime and/or wake time around), a teen's sleeping late in the morning, not having sunlight in the morning, or napping. Another reason is that he does not have enough wind-down time or a bedtime routine, and he has been exposed to light and mental stimulation too close to bedtime, not giving his body time to relax and release melatonin to prepare for sleep. See the Five Habits of Happy Sleepers in chapter 6 for help adjusting these factors.

My teen sleeps from about 11:30 p.m. to 6:30 a.m., but she says she feels fine.

Many adolescents don't complain about feeling sleep deprived, even though they are. This could be because they're more resilient and flexible than we adults are, but even if they don't feel tired, sleep deprivation takes its toll on mental health, metabolism, focus, decision-making, motivation, and more. Remember, we are not very accurate judges of our own sleep deprivation.

I go to bed and my son is still awake. How do I support him getting to sleep on time?

If you have a younger adolescent, we recommend establishing a regular, set bedtime and sticking to it. We find parents let go of good routines and sleep habits when their kids are too young (age twelve is when we see parents start to be hands-off on sleep habits). Remember, you are still in charge of such things. If you have an older teen approaching the end of high school, your approach will be different, because they should be taking over more control and decision-making when it comes to their sleep. Also, they have so much homework, you may really never be able to stay up as late as they do every night. Consider talking to your school about a homework limit (pointing out that excessive homework does not confer benefits), or talk to your teen and teachers about not complying with an arduous amount of homework if it seems unreasonable. In chapter 8 you will see examples of dialogue and ways to convey empathy, set limits, and help your teen find his self-motivation (page 225), which is key.

I think my son is just a night owl, and so am I. Are we just wired differently than morning people?

To some degree, yes. Preferences for evening and night versus morning is at least partially genetic—giving each of us a tendency toward our own natural rhythm as to when we feel most energetic and creative, and when we're ready to shut down. The reality is, though, that screens, phones, home lights, video games, work, and other forms of artificial light and activity suppress our body's natural rhythms. So a person with a slight night owl tendency can easily be swayed much later by habits and the environment. Since the world is, unfairly, geared toward morning people, it's usually the case that protecting wind-down routines and practicing the habits in chapter 6 become extra important to those who are geared as night owls.

4

Screens, Teens,
and the Missing Link

How many of these questions can you answer yes to?

Is your phone next to you while you're sleeping?
Do you check your phone when you wake in the middle of the night?
Do you work or do homework on a laptop in your bed?
Do you check social media or emails before you get out of bed in the morning?
Are you on a phone or tablet for most of the hour before bed?
Is your phone the last thing you see before you fall asleep, and the first thing you see in the morning?

Technology is thoroughly woven into our everyday lives. The Pew Research Center finds 95 percent of adolescents own or have exclusive access to a smartphone, and half say they're online on a near-constant basis. It may seem like a given that internet-enabled devices are all around us—in our hands, pockets, and backpacks, and within reach at every moment of the day. But this ubiquity is very new, especially for teenagers. In 2004, about half of teens had cell phones, but they were, well, phones—used for phone calls and simple text messages. Kids still commonly chatted with friends on the landline at home. The super-connected powers of the smartphone began to permeate teen life in 2008. By 2011, 23 percent of teens owned smartphones, in 2013 it was 37 percent, in 2014 it was 66 percent, and the most recent estimates are near complete saturation.

High-tech devices are also held by tinier and tinier hands. In 2015, 11 percent of eight-year-olds owned smartphones. Four years later, that had almost doubled, meaning that as of 2019, 1 in 5 third graders was carrying a small supercomputer in their backpacks. The vast majority of parents say they're concerned about the amount of time their child spends in front of a screen, and have asked for help and professional guidance to figure out what to do.

There's no doubt that smartphones, social media, gaming, and internet access have transformed daily life for most people on the planet. In our ongoing series of first-year parenting groups, the topic of screens is one of the most lively, as the moms and dads of eight-month-olds are already concerned about raising children in a digital age. They're presented with all forms of internet-enabled baby devices, debating at what age it's okay for kids to watch shows, and feeling bad about how their smartphones continually draw their attention away from their babies. Babies already see the phone as highly desirable. This object everyone is fascinated with must be.

It seems our parent instincts are right—there is cause for concern. Research indicates today's teenagers are struggling with more loneliness, depression, and anxiety, and more time spent on devices has been linked to this increase in mental health issues. Jean Twenge, a professor of psychology at San Diego State University, has analyzed some of the largest data sets on adolescents and has published widely on the behaviors of Gen Z. Her results point to an overall inverse relationship between time on digital media and well-being. For example, data gathered on half a million U.S. adolescents from grades 8 to 12 shows that, along with a significant increase in depressive symptoms and suicidal behaviors between 2010 and 2015 (when smartphone saturation spiked), more time on social media and smartphones was correlated with a higher likelihood of these and other mental health issues. In another analysis across three large data sets of U.S. and UK adolescents, Twenge and her colleagues found that measures of well-being and happiness were highest in "light" digital media users, and steadily declined with increasing hours spent texting, on social media, and gaming. Risk factors for self-harm followed the same pattern, with light users having the least risk, increasing thereafter toward heavy users, who had the highest risk. The percentage of adolescents reporting low well-being increased by 25 percent with each additional hour of average daily time online. Heavy users of social media were 83 percent more likely to say they were unhappy than light users.

All of this is concerning, which is why screens are such a hot topic for us parents. We have ongoing conversations about how to help kids navigate technology. Websites and bookstores are full of helpful writing on the subject.

But there is a missing link in this story about technology and teenagers—a force at play that is vastly underappreciated. This missing link helps us explain the connection between heavy technology use, depression, anxiety, and other negative outcomes. And the best news is that, whereas fighting technology as a whole can feel like swimming against the tide (impossible), this link is something you absolutely *do* have control over, and if you protect it, you also protect kids from the worrisome consequences of excessive screen time. If you've guessed it already, you know us too well by now. Yes, it's sleep.

Research links high levels of screen time to negative outcomes like poor mood, behavioral issues, unhealthy eating, and so forth. But if you read the fine print, many studies of screen use also detect a loss of sleep as a side effect. For example, a study of Chinese students found that excessive mobile phone use was linked to mental distress, but it was also linked to shorter weekday sleep and excessive daytime sleepiness.

Let's refresh our memory on the consequences of too little sleep: negative mood, low impulse control, lack of motivation, unhealthy eating, emotional fragility—it sounds suspiciously similar to those of heavy screen time, doesn't it? That's because heavy screen use disrupts sleep, which leads to the long and all-too-familiar list of issues teens face every day.

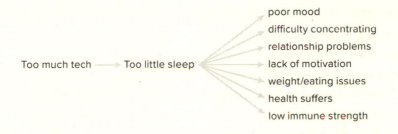

Too much tech ⟶ Too little sleep

- poor mood
- difficulty concentrating
- relationship problems
- lack of motivation
- weight/eating issues
- health suffers
- low immune strength

Lost sleep is a devastating consequence of too much technology. This often gets glossed over because sleep is seen as optional and dispensable, and because most people don't realize how the hour of sleep they or their teen misses is critical to their brain and body. What's great is that, in addition to all the mental and physical health benefits of good sleep we've explored, sleeping well can actually break an unhealthy technology cycle: a recent study by researchers at the University of Oregon found that young teens, ages twelve to fourteen, who spent less time on electronics before bed had more sleep and less daytime sleepiness, but it also found that this made them less susceptible to subsequent screen use. More sleep feeds kids with the protective nutrients they need to ward off the negative effects of technology: it gives kids better impulse control, more energy for physical activity, a more optimistic outlook, more curiosity, and more patience to figure out real-world problems. All of this helps them feel motivated to spend a healthier balance of their time offline.

FROM DARKNESS, TO THE LIGHTBULB, TO THE SMARTPHONE

Sleep protects our teens, but technology never stops chasing them. The incentive for technology companies is to keep teens engaged and connected, and these advances never stop. From basic video games to enchanting algorithms that mimic gambling, to constant alerts and prompts, to absorbing virtual reality headsets—electronic media is breathtaking in how good it is, and therefore how hard it is to put down. This means we have to understand how technology impacts sleep, and then learn the habits that keep healthy boundaries around it, so it doesn't hijack our finely tuned sleep systems. We can't go back to the days of lanterns and checkers (and we wouldn't want to—we love to watch our favorite shows like everyone else), but smart technology habits are absolutely in our grasp, and developing them as a family will raise our quality of life.

PARENTAL INVOLVEMENT MAKES A DIFFERENCE

When it comes to sleep, parents have more influence than they think. Research shows a high correlation between parent and teen sleep habits, which means that parents who prioritize their sleep are more likely to have teens who do too. As kids get older, parents often loosen expectations around sleep, and this leads the hours of sleep to go down. But research has shown that if parents stay involved—by setting and maintaining bedtimes—this effect is minimized. Importantly, in a few of these studies, parental involvement was found to be most powerful for kids who use their cell phones a lot in the evening before bed. Meaning kids who are heavy tech users around bedtime are the ones who most need their parents' input and help.

Let's back up a hundred years or so, to give ourselves and our teens a heavy dose of empathy for the predicament we're in. In the context of human history, the influx of light, in and of itself, is a very recent phenomenon: the lightbulb was introduced just before the turn of the twentieth century. For hundreds of thousands of years previously, humans slept with natural cues of darkness and light. That means human evolution is entirely set to the backdrop of the daily rising and setting sun. From the lightbulb to the smartphone to the present day is a tiny blip in the human time scale. This is why, when it comes to basic human functions like sleep, our brains are easily confused and overwhelmed. The prehistoric sleep systems in our brains developed to follow sunset, sunrise, temperature, and nature sounds, not electronic lights, YouTube, and social media alerts.

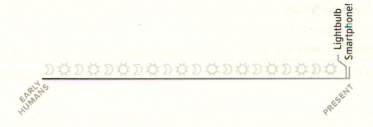

The lightbulb and technological advances like televisions and computers have had a significant effect on human sleep. Since their advent, we've been able to stay awake during the biological night, and healthy sleep has been on the decline as a result. But the internet and the smartphone have taken this decline into a nosedive. Between 2012 and 2015, the number of teens sleeping less than seven hours a night jumped by 22 percent. Again, researcher Jean Twenge, who analyzed this data, noted that while factors like time spent on homework, work, and extracurricular activities stayed relatively constant during this period, what did change drastically is that the majority of teens owned smartphones.

So why exactly does technology impact adolescent sleep? It's important to understand the mechanisms so we can help our teens make changes that restore healthy sleep. Here are the sleep-stealing routes technology takes:

Sleep chemistry is suppressed. As we learned in the previous chapter, light, including artificial light, suppresses the release of melatonin, the body's sleep-promoting chemical. Remember that after the sun goes down, our bodies interpret what should be the lack of light as a signal that it's time to settle in and allow the natural waves of sleep to take over. Light—from screens and lightbulbs—tricks the body and keeps us in an alert, awake state, in which we're no longer in touch with our body's natural clock–induced signals. All of these sources of light detract from our paleo-sleep. The most sleep-suppressing light is shorter wavelength light, which is blue (versus longer wavelength light, which is red). Home lights and screen lights often contain a lot of blue light.

We all suffer from this dilemma, but adolescents are the most affected because they are closely tied to their screens, and because of the biological factors we learned about in the previous chapter: the circadian rhythms shift later; the pressure to sleep builds more slowly, so teens have a higher tolerance for staying up; and they become especially sensitive to the alerting effects of light. Adolescent melatonin is easily suppressed. All of this makes adolescents more prone to delayed sleep, and technology seizes on this. A teen who might naturally go to bed at 10:00 p.m. can be pushed to 1:00 a.m. by the light of technology. This is true of home lights as well; lights in the house compound with the light from our devices to delay sleep.

A study of Italians during the pandemic lockdowns found that 90 percent increased their electronic device usage during that time, and this was tied to later bedtimes, later rise times, poorer sleep quality, and less sleep overall.

Emotions and thoughts are stirred. It's not just light that keeps our brains awake at night, it's all the mental stimulation that technology offers: the possibilities, realizations, frustration, curiosity, creative inspiration, sadness, excitement, and all the other alerting brain exercises that social media, games, and the internet deliver around the clock. Evolutionarily, the human brain is not equipped to handle this constant excitement. Fight-or-flight signals tell us not to sleep if there's a mystery to solve or danger around the corner, and these millennia-old brain circuits cannot tell the difference between real drama and threats and screen-generated ones. Are we running from a saber-toothed tiger in real life or are we just trying to defeat the game's enemy? Either way, the brain tells us to keep going, not to sleep.

Anxiety can be a particularly acute sleep stealer. Anxiety creeps into many people's sleep (and unfairly, lack of sleep then contributes to anxiety). For a teen, it might be worries over friendships, pressure created by academic expectations, financial strain, physical safety, and more. The same worries plague adults of course. During the pandemic, as we saw so many lose jobs and loved ones and basic security, anxiety levels rose. In our sleep-consulting practice, we started to hear more parents say, "You helped my baby/child sleep, but now I'm the one who's not sleeping." There isn't a simple fix for anxiety, but we know that interventions that reduce financial stress and uncertainty make families feel more secure, which leads to better sleep. We have to feel safe to sleep well.

When it comes to trying to disconnect and calm the mind before sleep, the key is to relax, distract, or "bore" our busy brain to the degree that it feels safe and calm enough to let sleep take over. That feeling of safety and relative boredom is actually very important at promoting sleep. The Five Habits of Happy Sleepers, which you will learn in chapter 6, will help you create the sleep bubble—adding to your sense of safety and relaxation. The "passive distractions" on pages 169–170 and the appendix tools can be particularly helpful for teens who find it very hard to wind down.

Just one more . . . We also lose sleep by what researchers call "displacement"—meaning that we simply spend time on gadgets and screens when we would otherwise be sleeping. We watch another episode, get to another level, or investigate another question. We get pulled

PANDEMIC SLEEP AND TECHNOLOGY

The pandemic was an interesting experiment in adolescent sleep in many ways. A group, including Kenneth Wright, Horacio de la Iglesia (whose work we discussed in chapter 3), and UC Boulder researcher Céline Vetter, compared the sleep of undergrad students at the University of Colorado Boulder at the beginning of 2020 before the stay-at-home orders to their sleep patterns later in the year. During stay-at-home, the students went to bed later, had thirty minutes more sleep on average, and experienced reduced social jet lag between weekday and weekend sleep. Anecdotally, parents of middle and high schoolers shared mixed experiences with us. One theme early in the pandemic was that teenagers were sleeping more, and their sleep shifted later, in line with their natural rhythms. Parents and teens shared relief and reduced morning stress without having to commute. As the year went on, we heard more and more stories of extremely late bedtimes, heavy technology use, teens spending a lot of time in their bedrooms (with disrupted daily rituals, reduced sun, and little signal to their circadian clocks), higher stress, and in some cases, less sleep. Indeed, a survey conducted by the nonprofit Challenge Success found that in the fall of 2020, the average twelfth grader was sleeping only 6.4 hours per night. Twenty-three percent of those surveyed said they were sleeping more than pre-pandemic, while 43 percent said they were sleeping less.

In other words, the pandemic was a mixed bag for sleep, but one of the takeaways was that increased anxiety and increased technology use may have decreased sleep for many teens. We can find ways to counteract the pandemic-induced heavy reliance on screens. Wherever possible, schools can swap device-delivered assignments and reading for textbooks and good old-fashioned paper printouts (have students hand them back at the end of the month so they can be reused). Less screen time equals better posture (have you noticed a slight slump in your teen's back?), better eating habits, more family conversations. Oh, and did we mention, better sleep?

down a river of content, and time passes. We cruise right past our bedtime, waving to it on the shores as the current of technology pulls us along. We are far past our ideal bedtime by the point we finally shut technology down. As the night goes on and we're up past our bedtimes, our rational decision-making ability goes down, we lose good judgment, and we stay up even later.

Technology creates "flow." The displacement theory is gaining a lot of ground as a powerful route by which technology decreases sleep. And there is a reason that people are spending more and more time on technology (and less time on sleep) than they ever did before. Game design and algorithms are getting better at keeping us in a state of flow. Flow is an experience of immersion in an activity, in which time is distorted and goes by without us having an accurate sense of it passing. Has your teen ever ex-

THE PSYCHOLOGICAL AND NEUROCHEMICAL POWER OF GAMES

In case this was up for debate, game developers do not seem to have our teens' sleep and mental health in mind. Quite the opposite, they purposefully design games that wield neurochemical power to keep kids coming back. Through no fault of their own, kids crave the dopamine-releasing stimulation built into social media and games. The level of intentional brain domination on the part of developers and companies in some cases qualifies as downright malevolent. Certain mobile games that seem innocuous and kid-friendly are essentially gambling games in disguise, and therefore dangerous for kids who can be roped into their addiction model. In-game purchases, randomized "loot boxes" with unknown prizes in them, intermittent rewards that are frontloaded and then begin to dwindle and give the child the sense of "Just one more and I'll get the prize!"—these games are built with intentionally addictive algorithms. This has been aptly called "weaponized behavioral psychology."

claimed, "I *just* got on!" after spending two hours playing a video game? This is flow, and some kids seem to be more prone to it. Researcher Mike Gradisar at Flinders University in Australia has been digging into the mechanisms by which technology affects adolescent sleep for many years.

SIGNS YOUR TEEN MIGHT NEED OUTSIDE HELP

Many of us know we have less-than-ideal technology habits. Maybe we automatically turn to our devices without conscious thought, allow news alerts to be fed to us through social media instead of purposely looking for news from our trusted sources, get emotionally triggered by various platforms and content, or sometimes feel bound to our phones. However, when we take a trip and leave the devices behind or break the habit in another way, we feel better. For some, this quick "reset" is not so easy, though. High levels of addiction that markedly lower a person's quality of life, decrease basic functioning, draw them away from real-life experiences, impair their relationships, severely impact sleep, and are very resistant to change often require professional treatment. If your teen falls into this category, it's best to seek immediate help by asking your pediatrician or some other trusted expert for a referral. Here are some signs you might need to check in with a professional. Your teen is:

- Absorbed or obsessed with the internet and spends excessive hours throughout the day
- Showing symptoms of anxiety, depression, or irritability when devices are gone
- Having academic problems, disengaged from or sleeping in class
- Less interested in the pastimes they used to enjoy and repeatedly choosing to spend time online rather than with friends or hobbies
- Covering up or lying about use
- Turning to the internet to escape from negative emotions
- Ignoring personal hygiene

His work suggests that some teens are more prone to becoming engrossed and experiencing flow, and this may contribute significantly to their decision to keep going, not to turn off games, and to delay sleep. He estimates that "the biggest influence is when a vulnerable person (with certain personality traits, like flow) falls victim to the greedy intentions of tech companies."

SMARTPHONES ARE THE NEW TEDDY BEARS

Now that we know how technology interferes with sleep, we can see why sharing a room with our devices is problematic. Still, most of us do. Three-quarters of all children and nearly 90 percent of adolescents have at least one device in their sleep environment, with most used near bedtime. More than a third of middle and high schoolers say they wake up at least once a night to check notifications or interact on their phone. We've talked to many teens who place their phones on their pillow to sleep, or just fall asleep while texting and never intentionally put their phones down.

Not surprisingly, abundant studies link poor sleep to screen use. Teens who have a device on after bedtime get nearly an hour less sleep than their peers with no electronics on at night. In fact, the presence of media devices in the bedroom (even without use) is associated with worse sleep. This screen-sleep relationship is true of the littlest kids: preschool-age children who watch more TV in the evening or have a TV in their room sleep less overall and are more likely to have a sleep problem. A study of Thai infants even found that those who were exposed to screen media after 7:00 p.m. slept a half hour less than infants with no evening screen exposure. A review of sixty-seven articles between 1999 and 2014 looking at TV, computers, video games, and mobile devices found that more screen time overall, and more evening screen time in particular, meant less sleep and later sleep. In this review, 76 percent of the studies found a link between TV watching and less sleep, but 94 percent found a significant link between computer or internet use and how much sleep adolescents got. In one study, those who said they usually or always used the internet for social reasons at bedtime got fifty-one minutes less sleep than their peers—which is a large chunk of a whole sleep cycle. One study of middle schoolers found that an hour more screen time in the evening was associated with more than a threefold risk of going to bed at 10:00 p.m. or later. A recent study of university students in the UK found that those who used their phones late at night were three times as likely to have problematic or "addictive" phone behavior and poorer sleep. A study of French adolescents found that sleep-deprived teens were more likely to have devices in their bedrooms, and that feelings of sadness and irritability were more common in sleep-deprived teens. Need we go on?

South Korea, where high school students routinely sleep only five or six hours a night, is one of the most wired countries in the world, and researchers have found that, for these kids, more screen use is linked to less sleep, as well as poorer academic performance and more mental health issues. With so many hours per day dedicated to school, study, and screens, it's not surprising that 95 percent of Korean teens report insufficent physical activity, and a third said they don't exercise at all except in physical education classes at school. In fact, Korean doctors are seeing dramatic cases of teens seeking professional help for screen addiction. "Addiction camps" are trying to help teenagers unplug and regain their sleep and mental and physical health. Health experts in Korea have warned that if the U.S. doesn't act, this public health crisis is coming for it next. In a move to buffer kids' mental and physical health, China enacted regulations around video games: kids under eighteen can only play for an hour a day on Fridays, weekends, and holidays.

What all of this means is that technology is a powerful but often silent sleep stealer—delaying and disrupting teen sleep through multiple routes—and lost sleep is one of the least appreciated links between technology and teen mental health. Sleeping thirty to sixty minutes less decreases activity in the prefrontal cortex, which means kids can't think as clearly or pay proper attention in school, and they are more likely to make bad decisions. Their sharp focus is dulled and creative problem-solving is limited. Losing this hour of sleep amps up our kids' emotional brains, and leaves them more likely to feel stressed, anxious, and pessimistic about the world.

The force of technology can feel overwhelming to us as parents—something that showed up on our doorstep, unannounced. We don't remember swinging the door wide open and welcoming it inside. Or at least we thought we'd be able to tell it when to leave. But it now seems like a permanent houseguest—both loved and hated. Knowing that technology affects our kids' sleep and health can feel unfair and frustrating: Why do tobacco, vaping, or drug companies have to acknowledge responsibility when marketing and selling to teens, but technology companies have absolutely no regulation in offering and hooking kids? Big tech seems to have a free pass with our teens.

We do have the power to use our devices in a way that we choose rather than a way chosen for us. Setting boundaries around this ever-evolving force is in our control and will be one of the most powerful ways to protect our kids' sleep, health, and happiness.

PRACTICAL STEPS:
SPOTTING YOUR "SLEEP STEALERS"

Home lights, tablets, televisions, phones, and computers—all have the ability to delay and disrupt sleep, for the reasons we have outlined. The brighter-light, closer-held devices and those that emit blue light are more likely to suppress melatonin and delay sleep. Entertainment that is interactive, emotionally charged, dramatic, interesting, or opens up more questions will keep us up longer through stirring emotions and also through displacement, or may simply cause us to be awake when our bodies would otherwise be asleep. Video games can keep us in a flow state.

For these reasons, changing your screen habits is one of the most powerful ways to improve sleep. In chapter 6, you'll read more about your sleep stealers and your three routines, including wind-down, bedtime, and morning routines, but for our purposes here, it's important to say that screens are the main factor to change during routines in order to promote healthy sleep. A recent study of adolescents, for example, found that instructing them to put away their phones one hour before bed, for one week, led to them shutting down devices earlier, turning off the lights earlier, and sleeping more.

This is because sleep starts before you get into bed, which is an un-derappreciated fact. The opening act to sleep starts about an hour or two before you lie down, as your internal clock strikes its wind-down hour and your sleep chemistry emerges from behind the curtain. But screens interfere with this opening act—delaying the show by hours sometimes. Protecting sleep means protecting the prelude to sleep. This prelude is your wind-down time. During wind-down time, here is an example of dos and don'ts:

SCREEN DOS	SCREEN DON'TS
Watch a movie (passive)	Play video games (interactive)
Watch TV on a television (distant)	Watch a TV show on a laptop (close)
Read with red color reading light	Read with bright lights on

(Read more dos and don'ts on page 159.)

Entertainment that is passive, such as watching a movie, is less likely to amp up your body chemistry than being on social media or watching YouTube videos that send the viewer down a rabbit hole of content. These interactive activities introduce questions, puzzles, or worries to our brain late at night: *Can I get to the next level? I'm not sure I can make that deadline...Am I going to get a good grade? I better think more about this... What are my friends doing right now?* They prompt us to keep going rather than disconnecting to let our bodies fall asleep.

Music is often used as a sleep aid, but to the surprise of many of our clients, music listening has been linked to poorer sleep. There are a few reasons that listening to music may not be a good idea as an activity while falling asleep. Music can be too interesting and stir emotions that make it hard to become drowsy—after all, music is emotional by its very nature. Music is often played from a device that also has access to the internet, games, messages, and more, so listening to music is a gateway to the rest of the world. Finally, if we fall asleep or get very sleepy with music playing and then it turns off, the change can confuse and disorient

---

PRACTICAL TEEN TIP:
GET YOUR DAILY DOSE OF "VITAMIN C"

One of the reasons teens are glued to their phones and sleep with them on their pillows is that the connection to friends is so important. When teens are missing time to hang out in a small friend group and just chill, the phone becomes a lifeline. And even though studies show that social media is a poor alternative to this need, if by the evening that need is not filled, they are hungry for it. Protecting some downtime with what psychologist Ron Taffel calls the "second family" is important, and filling up on this in-person time makes it easier to say goodbye and turn the phone off at a reasonable hour. Hanging out after school or mid-evening before dinner is like taking a dose of vitamin C, for Connection. When Julie's son was in high school, they had a finished garage, which gave him space to hang with friends. When he was a younger teen, she would show up at the door when the pizza arrived or for any reason. As he got older, she stopped showing up unannounced. It was hard but clear that he needed that space and for her to trust him and his friends.

WHERE IS THE RESPONSIBLE DESIGN?

It's important to reiterate that screen behaviors and habits that interfere with sleep are not parents' or teens' fault. Many parents tell us they feel guilty or bad for not better managing their child's screen time. But technology companies and individuals design games and media that are *purposefully* engineered to hook and consume our kids. It's not our own weakness or fault (or our kids')—social media and other digital platforms are designed to tap into our brain's reward systems, and kids are especially vulnerable. Entrepreneur and philanthropist Andrew Yang, who has two kids, aptly writes: "Right now, the interests of parents are directly at odds with the interests of the technology companies. They're monetizing our attention and profiting off of our time. As they say, the addictive nature of smartphones is a feature, not a bug." He recommends regulating simple features like autoplay on children's media, which does not allow a natural end to a show but feeds endless content to kids on platforms like Netflix and YouTube. Tristan Harris, a former Google designer, who many will remember from the movie *The Social Dilemma*, describes how social networks and websites measure success in clicks, swipes, and time spent online, not by the positive value they add to people's lives. He points out that companies and designers absolutely have the power to change this, and users (parents) can demand that technology is built around adding value. Rather than feeling as though we're failing as parents, we should put the onus back on companies for responsible design—especially when it comes to kids and teens. Vote for representatives and politicians who talk about this issue and have specific ideas for responsible measures and for how to incentivize responsible design. Buy and support platforms and games that do add value and allow parents and teens to better monitor and manage their use. Media companies like Netflix and YouTube should give parents of young kids the ability to create a playlist that includes only the shows the parents choose and does not suggest and link to a multitude of others (which, again, all have autoplay and keep endlessly running). It needs to be easier for parents and kids to choose what they want to see and not be bombarded afterward.

This is a really helpful insight to share with kids, to make them smart consumers. Tell your kids that algorithms, tech companies, social media platforms, and more are designed to hook and keep them—for money. When kids are empowered with this knowledge, it can help them develop a healthier relationship to technology. You can say, "YouTube would absolutely *love* for you to be awake all night."

the brain later in the night (when the music is no longer there) and wake us up. For teens who need help winding down, quieting their minds, and falling asleep, we recommend a meditation or relaxation tool (see the appendix), and if that's not working, passive distractions (page 169). Done the right way, music *can* be a passive distraction. Read more about passive distractions to see if music listening is the right choice, or if there's a better way to relax before bed.

FAMILIES WHO ARE *F-O-N-D* OF EACH OTHER

Okay, parents, here's where we look to ourselves, because how we manage our devices sets a healthy (or unhealthy) example for our teens. It's harder to make the case for kids not having technology in the bedroom and in the sleep routines (as we'll help you accomplish in chapter 6) if as parents we don't follow our own advice. Little kids and teenagers model their behaviors (often subconsciously) after their parents, so if your phone is an appendage and your attention is continually drawn to it, this behavior pattern is more likely to be adopted by your kids. When you practice basic boundaries and good screen habits, this also rubs off on the whole family. Not only that, it signifies to your teen that your own sleep and well-being are a priority.

Parents have room for improvement in this arena. The majority of parents say they sleep with a mobile device next to their bed, and about 1 in 4 say they wake up to check their phone in the night. If you ask children about their parents' screen behaviors, many will express disdain for the phone and say their mom or dad is always on it and it's hard to get their attention. Half of adolescents say their parent or caregiver is distracted by their cell phone when they're trying to have a conversation with them.

Most parents are aware that babies and little kids need our attention, but we don't appreciate how much teenagers do too. They pick up on signs of distraction, like when our eyes are glued to a screen, when it takes many attempts to get our attention, or when we pick up our phones in every down moment as if the device is more interesting than the moment in front of us. It's a huge relief to kids when we watch and listen. It makes them feel seen, validated, and understood. This is not just something we save for a big moment of "Hey, Mom, I need to talk to you." Rather, teens pick up on our nuanced distraction all the time. In addition, if you regularly talk, text, and type in destinations on your phone while you're driving, your teen won't take you seriously when you tell him how dangerous distracted driving is.

The irony is that parents are much more likely to turn to their phone when a child is acting out or a teen is nonresponsive or withdrawn, creating a further breakdown in communication when they need us most. In these difficult moments, it's easier to retreat to our corners and not deal with what's going on under the surface. It makes perfect sense that our instinct is to distract ourselves from the reality of how hard these moments can feel, but as we grow the habit of escaping to our screens, we get rustier and rustier at effective communication with our kids. By not giving up and turning to your devices, you are refusing to be influenced by a force, created by technology, that is carrying you further and further from your teen.

The antidote to this powerful pull of technology is twofold. One, healthy screen habits (which we will help you establish at the end of this chapter and in chapter 6), and two, the broader family elements that lead to greater well-being, connection, and sleep. We think of these elements like daily vitamin doses that keep everyone *F-O-N-D* of each other:

Family rituals. Teenagers grow more independent, but they continue to need the primary attachment to family. As kids get older, it's important to protect the rituals of dinner together, movie night, Sunday-morning hikes or throwing a baseball, bedtime routines, and so forth. Rituals are different from spontaneous times together (which are important too) because they are predictable and lead to a feeling of belonging and security. Too often we see families grow disconnected from each other while living under the same roof, and this is accentuated by electronic media. Remember the data mentioned earlier in the chapter on U.S. middle and high school kids' screen time and mental health? That data found that those kids who spent more time on *non*-screen activities, like in-person social interactions, sports or exercise, print media, and attending religious services, were less likely to have mental health issues. These real-world routines and rituals have clear benefits and help our kids grow a healthy sense of self, purpose, and connection to our family and community.

Open play. Play is an intrinsic human drive, and it's essential to the brain. Through play, kids learn to solve problems, stretch creativity, sustain attention, and feel joy, satisfaction, and accomplishment. The trouble is that play (of the non-digital variety) can easily disappear as kids get older. Most people know that little kids need to play, but as they mature, we respect this need less and less. Psychologist Stuart Brown has researched play for decades, finding many connections between play (at all ages) and our happiness and fulfillment as individuals, resilience, flexibility, and connection to one another as social beings. "Nothing lights up the brain like play," says Brown. What constitutes play is that it's done for enjoyment and exploration (not necessarily an organized sport). Building a

PARENTS AND THE "STILL FACE" STUDY

In the 1970s, researchers devised the Still Face paradigm to show a fundamental dynamic between babies and parents. In the experiment, the parent goes from engaging, smiling, talking to, and making eye contact with the baby to keeping their face expressionless and unresponsive. They are physically there, but emotionally flat. Within minutes, the baby quickly goes from chatting and exploring the room to being stressed, dysregulated, and no longer interested in the environment.

Recently, this experiment has been replicated, but instead of being expressionless, the parent is on a mobile device. The results were almost identical. The infants' stress levels increased. They became less curious and took more time to recover emotionally when the mothers put their devices down and shifted their attention back to their babies.

Similarly, as parents, when we are repeatedly distracted by our phones or other devices, being physically present while psychologically absent can negatively impact our relationship with our kids and our ability to communicate effectively. Parents know that teens need more space and independence, but it's too easy to throw up our hands and overdo it by allowing each person to go into their own electronic world. When we're on our devices, we miss subtle cues from our kids, and the allure of screens can make it seem easier to keep the peace in the short term, while risking missing out on valuable opportunities to communicate. When we put down devices and make eye contact, respond with empathy, and protect face-to-face family time, it helps to build trust, connection, and enjoyment of each other's company that are key to well-being. This essential need doesn't end just because our kids are a little older.

model robot, finding random materials to make a hangout spot, climbing a hill and rolling down, or just riding bikes around the neighborhood are examples. "The opposite of play is not work," says Brown. "It's depression."

Play is a component of happiness, and it leads our kids, teens, and us as adults to feel better regulated, connected, and healthier. It's basically an antidepressant and should be protected as kids get older. Play—especially outdoors—improves our sleep. What's amazing is how natural the drive is to play, so promoting it does not have to be fancy at all. All you need is the opportunity for play: time and space away from screens. When kids are together, without screens, they play together instinctively (as they get older, they just need a little warm-up time). Don't worry about the complaints about boredom or the resistance to getting outside. With time, the drive to play takes over.

Nature. Being in nature has been found to lower levels of stress hormones (which also helps us sleep), increase cognitive abilities, and improve mood. One study found that gardening for thirty minutes significantly reduced stress chemicals, even more than reading for the same amount of time. Another found that walking in nature reduced activity in the part of the brain responsible for rumination (continuously thinking about something that bothers you). Sunlight early in the day stimulates the brain to become alert, increases mood-improving neurochemicals, and deepens our sleep in the forthcoming night.

Remember Max, from the previous chapter? One of the main factors that led to the disappearance of his seemingly entrenched sleep issues was the sheer amount of time he spent outside when he went to camp. Sunlight (even through clouds), fresh air, and the visual elements and colors of nature stimulate the brain, reducing stress and syncing us with our body's natural rhythms.

Downtime. If every moment of your day is accounted for, there is no opportunity to become bored, or have a new idea or a spontaneous experience that isn't pre-scripted. Downtime is easily squeezed by busy family life, but we find it helps everyone feel better when there's some downtime built into each week. It sounds counterintuitive to schedule downtime, but that's what most families need to do, and it works well.

The combination of healthy screen habits and *F-O-N-D* family elements improves sleep by feeding family connection, fun, and meaning, as well as keeping us in control of our devices so we can enjoy their benefits and then put them away.

⌣

PRACTICAL TAKEAWAYS FOR FAMILIES: MEETINGS AND FAMILY AGREEMENTS

Family meetings are a really helpful practice. Rather than waiting for a problem and then calling a family meeting, which naturally gives a negative tone to the meeting, see if you can have regular family meetings, every week, or at least every month, so that creative ideas can be shared and solutions worked on. The idea is not to fight fires with family meetings but to prevent them in the first place.

What is the goal of family meetings?

To come up with family agreements
To give everyone in the family a chance to express feelings and ideas and to feel heard
To foster a sense of connection
To talk about what's working well and what still needs problem-solving
To talk about fun family plans (outings, trips, events, etc.)

Here are some guidelines for family meetings:

Involve everyone in the family, even very young children.
Try having one person (child or parent) "run" the meeting. This person can decide the format. Any format is fine, as long as every person has the opportunity to talk. Try not to have parents run the meeting every time.
Give everyone a chance to share. Only one person should talk at a time. Resist talking over one another, correcting, or adding your thoughts while another person is talking. Wait until the person

is done and see if you can summarize what they said. Ask if you've got it right.

Choose someone (child or parent) to be the note taker.

Parents, if you have an issue or complaint to bring up, try starting with the words "I've noticed..."

See how this changes the message:

Instead of:

Your video games are a problem. I've told you a million times to turn them off and you don't listen to me. I'm going to have to take them away if you don't learn.

Say:

I've noticed you're really interested in video games these days, and it seems hard to turn them off, even when we've agreed on it.

Instead of:

You are really on bad behavior these days. You've been mean to your sister. She isn't doing anything wrong and you're just rude all the time.

Say:

I've noticed you have a really harsh tone with your sister this week. Can you tell us more about what's going on?

Come up with family agreements during your meetings. You don't have to form all your family agreements at once—it can be a list that takes a few meetings to form. Agreements are what you'd think of as "rules," but the spirit is collaborative and everyone can contribute ideas to form this list.

HOW TO CHANGE HABITS: HARNESSING THE POWER OF THE SUBCONSCIOUS

In a relative blip on the human time scale, electronic media has transformed our daily habits and behaviors. Checking our phones, texting, looking at updates—much of this behavior is done automatically, without conscious thought. Our hands reach for our phones before our brains know why.

Changing our habits around screens is arguably the most profound and immediate way we can reclaim sleep. But how can you change your daily interactions with your screens? Actually, most of us have more control than we give ourselves credit for. We can change our screen behaviors and protect sleep with some simple habit-changing techniques.

People often assume willpower and determination are the answers to changing habits, but it turns out that habits are largely subconscious and automatic. We don't think about each step; we just float through without attention or focus. Once we've picked up our phone to check on incoming messages or alerts hundreds, thousands of times, that behavior has become automatic, below the level of conscious decision.

Tech companies are all too familiar with our subconscious tendencies, and they take advantage of this knowledge. Just like fast-food restaurants hook us with bright colors and tons of salt, our phones use pings and red alerts, streaming services instantly start the next episode, and algorithms know how to serve us more and more provocative or controversial content that we easily lose hours watching. Video games are brilliantly designed to keep us climbing levels and gathering rewards. In all cases, it's the companies' goal for us to become addicted to our devices. It certainly isn't a coincidence that most of us are.

Social psychologist Wendy Wood calls a habit "a mental shortcut" and explains that successful people often get to where they are in life by setting themselves up for good habits. Knowing we've been sucked in and being determined to change isn't enough, because the subconscious makes us do things without thinking in the first place. In other words, consciously changing *bad* habits isn't as effective as making *good* habits subconscious. Since our screen behaviors affect our sleep to a huge degree and are largely habitual, it makes sense to learn a few strategies for better managing these habits in our daily lives.

Tweak your environment. Setting your teen up for success can be as easy as showing them how to make tweaks to the environment. The goal is to decrease friction for new desired habits while increasing friction for old undesired habits. For example, when students study in the library (instead of a dorm room with a TV) and fill their fridges with healthy foods, their diet, sleep, and study habits improve. Situational variables can dramatically increase our ability to do the thing we want to do. In fact, Wendy Wood points out that there was a little-known aspect of the famous "marshmallow experiment," in which little kids who exerted greater control over eating the fluffy white treat showed discipline that later was linked to success in life: the kids were able to wait longer if the marshmallow was hidden.

What you can do: Increase friction for old "bad" habits

- Put your phone on a bookshelf or in some other out-of-the-way location (keep the ringer on but alerts off).
- Close your computer and put it away in a drawer or behind a closed door if possible when work or homework is done.
- Put your video game headset in a cabinet instead of on the coffee table.
- Charge your phone at night in a room that is not your bedroom.
- Unless you need it, put your phone in the back seat of the car or in the trunk so it's more likely you'll turn the radio on or talk to your passenger. This is also a safe driving practice for parents and teens.

(continued)

What you can do: Decrease friction for new "good" habits

- Set an alert for when it's time to wind down.
- Buy or borrow an engrossing book and put it on your bedside table.
- Put board games and puzzles on an accessible shelf in the living room. Put Bingo or chess on the coffee table.
- Have your sneakers and outside clothes visible and ready to go, or even better, put them on when you get home from work or school.
- Ask your teen if she'd like to rearrange the furniture in her bedroom, add a sleep-friendly light, and maybe even paint the walls a different color. New, personally designed cues in the environment can make shifting to a new habit of going to bed at a regular, earlier time each night more alluring.
- Let your teen pick out an old-fashioned non-light-up alarm clock.
- Put a pad of paper, drawing utensils, and a pack of Sudoku in your bag and in the car. Heather makes sure to always have paper and writing utensils with her. Recently, her family was waiting for their dog in the parking lot outside the vet's office. Instead of turning to the automatic habit of getting on their phones, she and her son played word guessing games for thirty minutes.
- Set your phone on "Do not disturb" when you're working. Most phones have settings that allow you to choose your "favorite" people, whose calls and texts will still come through. Program specific ring tones for people you want to recognize. Set your phone to silence unknown callers.
- Find music, audiobooks, stand-up comedy, or podcasts that everyone likes to listen to in the car.

Over time, if you set up the environment in smart ways, eventually subconscious patterns emerge and good habits can take over.

Positively reinforce the new habit: We know that new habit formation improves when the new behavior is combined with or followed by a positive, associated experience. You are pairing a desired habit with something that feels good. Dopamine is released and the behavior is reinforced.

What you can do:

- Have healthy foods on hand for a pre-bedtime snack. Heather makes a plate of crackers, cheese, and sliced pears or apples to eat with her preteens while they watch a TV show before getting ready for bed.
- Stock up on simple, healthy breakfast foods your teen really likes. When she goes to bed in time to get up for breakfast, her favorite foods are right there, easy to grab. Put music on in the morning. Depending on whether she likes help and a morning chat, you can either be there or give her a little space as she wakes up.
- Decide on an interesting book series to read or listen to some soothing music or sounds after parking your phones at night. You can take turns reading a book out loud together or each person can read their own book silently. A family we know comes together at a certain time in the evening, with each person reading their own book.

Let the benefits of a good night's sleep be your teen's own "reward." Not every teen will report the delicious spring-in-our-step feeling we adults revel in after a good night's sleep, but over time, some will. Try to let the correlation between sleeping well and feeling good come from them. It's fine to ask an open-ended question like "How're you doing?" but refrain from asking, "Don't you feel good when you sleep well?" over and over. Let this be their discovery.

Change as a team. There is no doubt that we reduce friction for a new habit when we set common goals as a family or group. You can probably think of many ways your family has developed habits you enjoy by doing them together. Interconnected patterns emerge with activities like preparing and eating meals together, baking, attending community events, watching movies, playing

(continued)

games, even something as simple as tossing a ball. Studies around changing habits such as overeating show that people who live with healthy eaters have an easier time and more successful outcomes. Taking a sleep-forward approach as a family will be key to success. Think about setting a nightly time and place to charge everyone's phones (your teen can bust you if you don't adhere to it as well), helping one another set special alerts to signal wind-down time and shifting as a family to music, an audio-book, or watching a movie at an agreed-upon time. As your teen gets older and wants to be more independent, these family habits will influence her, even if you don't see it in the short term.

When people are tired, they're more likely to fall back on un-desired habits. This can create a cycle of bad sleep hygiene be-cause if we don't sleep well, we default to the easiest and most instantly gratifying thing. If you interrupt this cycle by consciously setting up the environment and creating good habits, your sleep will improve and you'll have more energy to put toward reinforcing those good habits.

Understanding the "below our awareness" aspect of habit for-mation in this way can help us be kinder to ourselves, which con-tributes to success and progress. When we can fine-tune our environments to create a smoother path for our new habits versus berating ourselves as failures for having no self-control, we avoid shutdown and resignation. It's liberating. These strategies will help as you create your Five Habits of Happy Sleepers in chapter 6 and pave the path to better sleep for the whole family.

FAMILY MEETING AGENDA ITEM: SCREENS

Not surprisingly, screens are a hot topic for family meetings. This is a good time to talk about phones, social media, games, and other forms of technology. Focus on creating a nonjudgmental tone in the meeting, or else you will engage the defenses of other family members and no understanding or solutions will come out of it. Here are to-dos for a family meeting on screens. (Note: Don't try to talk through these all at the same time; pick a few to start.)

1. **Pop quiz:** In our practice, we ask parents and kids these questions to evaluate how they're doing with screens (as they relate to sleep, daytime priorities, health, and well-being). This is not an official diagnostic tool, it's just our way of assessing whether families feel they have a healthy relationship with technology.

   Negative / Signs we have room for improvement

   - ☐ Do you look at your phone or computer within thirty minutes of your ideal bedtime?
   - ☐ Do you take your phone into your bedroom at night, with notifications on?
   - ☐ Do you look at your phone in the middle of the night, either because you've heard a notification or because you can't sleep?
   - ☐ Do you play video games or go online first thing in the morning?
   - ☐ Does social media feed you your news, or do you consciously look at trusted sources of news?
   - ☐ Do you feel down, anxious, or like you're missing out after scrolling social media?
   - ☐ Do you feel like your parents are distracted by their phones and computers?
   - ☐ Do you feel like something is missing (like a limb) if your phone isn't with you?
   - ☐ Are video games or phones a source of tension or arguments in your house?

Positive / Signs we are crushing it

Do you spend time outside every day? ☐

Do you exercise for at least half an hour every day, including ☐ activities like walking to school or work?

Are there non-screen based activities, like building, drawing, ☐ reading, experimenting or otherwise, that get you fired up? Do you dedicate enough, or as much time as you'd like, to those non-screen activities?

Do you have regular daily or weekly family rituals? Dinner to- ☐ gether, movie nights, walks outside, board games?

Count how many checks you have in the negative and positive categories and talk about it together.

2. **Learn together.** Choose a few interesting findings about sleep to highlight or that are aha moments. Adolescents like to understand their own brains and bodies, so we should trust and appeal to this inclination. It can be illuminating to discuss the financial motivations of big-tech companies and how they don't have our personal interests at heart. They just want to make money. Teens like having the insider, behind-the-scenes perspective.

3. **Create family agreements.** When teens have the information, they often make just as smart and wise decisions as parents about what's reasonable. Ask your teen what he thinks is a good amount of time each day on a particular app, and then work with him to set that time limit—you may be surprised that he has a great idea and a sense of this himself. Use one of the whiteboards you picked up during the pandemic to write notes. Decide on:

- Device-free zones and times. In these zones and times, it helps to put your phones in a designated place, like on a bookshelf, in a bag, or in a drawer. Device-free zones and times could include:

During meals (both in and out of the house)
An hour before bed
While driving or in the car in general, passenger or driver
During a conversation
For hellos and goodbyes (when your teen first gets home from
    school, while everyone is trying to leave the house, and so forth)
Don't text your teen when at school

- Screens-down time for weekdays and weekends. Ideally, this is thirty to sixty minutes before your bedtime. On the weekend, try to keep your screens-down time within one hour of your weekday time. Identify a location where everyone's phones and other devices will be after screens-down, until morning. You will learn more about this in chapter 6.

- Limits on particular apps or overall screen time. Decide together and set these up.

4. **Set up the environment and schedule for success.** We highly recommend the first three suggestions here.

- Turn off unnecessary notifications.

- Take TVs and computers (if possible) and other devices out of the bedroom. Having electronics in the bedroom is linked to worse sleep, so we advocate for not having them there at all. If you have a young adolescent (about age ten to fifteen), it's very reasonable (and we advise) having a phone-free bedroom. If you start with this rule and stick to it yourself, it's easier to maintain as time goes on. If that train has already left the station and you don't think it's possible to change course, refer to self-motivation on page 225.

- Buy a basic alarm clock with no lights for each person in the house who needs one.

- Try a daily "no screens" hour in addition to the hour before bed for two weeks. Or try a once-a-week "no screens" half day.

- For families with younger teens, try a time duration each day when everyone *can* use their screens. Parents, make sure to be transparent and honest about your allowed time for your computer or phone use. The precise and quantifiable changes in your habits are the ones that provide truly helpful modeling.

- Do a one-day-unplugged family challenge with a reward for those who make it and a "consequence" for those who don't (they have to do everyone's laundry or cook dinner three nights in a row).

- As a family, watch documentaries about this, such as *Screenagers* and *The Social Dilemma*.

A lot of parents tell us they've hit a wall when it comes to talking about screens and technology. They've tried to set rules, been stern, yelled, or pleaded, and eventually ended up feeling powerless and resentful and giving up. All these dynamics are understandable, but in the end, they make us feel more distant from each other. Parents in one room, kids in another, frustration around screens building. Screens may be here to stay, but our task as teens and parents is to use them in a smart way, and to be in control, rather than being controlled. We don't need to be pulled along a river of technology—we can decide when and where we go, and how we spend our time. With these solutions, we can better manage our electronics and protect healthy sleep for the whole family.

PRACTICAL STEPS FOR
SLEEP-FORWARD COMPANIES

Technology companies can take steps to make life better for users, especially kids. For example:

- Streaming platforms should give kids and parents a way to turn off autoplay functions, as well as "suggested" or "because you liked" functions. Netflix and others should allow you to create a playlist that is only chosen shows, that do not allow kids to hop to another unknown show with one tap.

- Make content delivery platforms and games have bedtimes. It should be easy for teens and parents to decide how long they'll play or watch something, to set an in-game or in-show timer, and to get a notification when that self-determined time is up.

- Game developers: Program in PSA-type messages that tell teens and parents it's time for winding down: "Your melatonin would like to emerge right now—are you ready to shut down?" The user might decide to play one more game or watch one more episode (don't tell anyone we suggested that), but at least it starts to nudge you in the right direction.

- In a genius design initiative, a Cornell Tech graduate student used principles of behavioral economics and psychology to develop an app that used negative reinforcement—in the form of persistent smartphone vibrations—to remind users they had exceeded their time limit on a certain app. Once they hit their predetermined limit, study participants' phones vibrated every five seconds until they navigated away. The reminder strategy reduced their time on Facebook—the chosen app for the study—by an average of 20 percent. Let's take this kind of example as inspiration and use our understanding of behavior for good, to promote messages for healthy screen use and healthy sleep.

5

Early Start Times and Academic Overload

One morning, Phyllis Payne was nursing her daughter in the pre-dawn hours. As it was still dark outside, she felt—as many parents of brand-new babies do—that she must be the only one awake. She looked out the window and saw a group of kids in backpacks milling through the dark. One of them was her babysitter.

When she asked about it later, the babysitter told her she and her high school classmates were waiting for the bus. It turned out that the local high schools in her county of Fairfax, Virginia, started at 7:20 a.m. Kids were getting up as early as 5:30 a.m. to get to school.

It seemed inhumane. Fairfax High School's students and their parents were complaining about the toll on kids' physical and mental health. Parents lamented sending their teens to school in the dark. Kids routinely fell asleep in class. One mom reported that her high-achieving son was taking allergy medication every night in a desperate attempt to help himself fall asleep, knowing he had to wake up at 5:50 a.m.

The Fairfax students were sleeping an average of 6.5 hours per night, and 20 percent were sleeping five hours or less on a regular basis. The mental and physical burden was overwhelming. The loss of sleep was linked to greater odds of feeling hopeless, seriously considering suicide, suicide attempts, and substance use.

To date, hundreds of studies have shown a pattern of increased mental health issues, decreased cognitive functioning, and a higher risk of car crashes associated with early school start times. And yet, as doctors, sleep experts, parent groups, students, and every major medical association make the case for change, early high school start times are the norm. Currently, almost half of U.S. public high schools start in the 7:00 a.m. hour, which means buses begin picking students up before 6:00 a.m., and some students have to wake up as early as 5:00 a.m. Given the average shift in the adolescent biological clock, this is equivalent to an adult waking every morning at 3:00 a.m.

How did this happen? And considering the health and well-being of our kids, what are we going to do about it?

THE HISTORY OF U.S. SCHOOL START TIMES

School schedules used to be reasonable. Older generations remember that school started around 8:30–9:00 a.m., and families often lived close, maybe even walked or biked to school. In the second half of the twentieth century, as the population grew and cities sprawled outward, schools and families grew farther apart and busing took on a greater and greater role. Bus fleets created a growing expense for school districts, so to manage

THE DECLINE OF WALKING TO SCHOOL

In 1969, 48 percent of students walked or biked to school.
In 2009, 13 percent of students walked or biked to school.

costs, schools created tiered systems of bus pickups in order to use the same buses for elementary, middle, and high schools—which required staggered schedules. In many districts, high school students were placed on the first tier. School officials thought they needed less sleep than younger students.

As a result, U.S. high school start times drifted earlier and earlier. In the 1960s, for example, Fairfax, Virginia, moved high schools to 8:15 a.m. and elementary schools to 8:45 a.m. to save on bus costs. In the 1970s, high school was shifted to 8:00 a.m. Already, parents were documented as complaining that this was too early, and that kids had to leave the house in the dark. By the mid-1980s, high schools in Fairfax started at 7:40 a.m., and by 1996, at 7:20 a.m.

Over recent decades, extremely early high school hours became the norm in the U.S., and during this time, teenage sleep deprivation slowly and surely became an accepted and normal fact of life. Many of us remember the feeling of having to peel ourselves out of bed way before our bodies were ready. Parents have always sensed something was wrong here—seeing their teens struggling to wake up and head out the door in a productive and positive mood, and trying desperately to make up for lost sleep on the weekends.

> *From Heather: I went to high school in the 1990s and remember winter mornings, standing at the bus stop as the sun was just coming up, and my hair had frozen!*

This exhaustion was confirmed by sleep science in the 1990s, as it became clear that there was a mismatch between school start times and adolescent biology. Beginning with the findings we explored in chapter 3, research clearly showed that adolescents need as much sleep or more than younger kids (and distinctly more sleep than adults). The intense period of adolescent brain construction was revealed. The delay in the circadian rhythms was uncovered. It started to dawn on scientists, clinicians, educators, and parents that teens were not magically making it all work with six to seven hours of sleep—they needed more like nine hours and were being pushed into extreme sleep deprivation. Mary Carskadon wrote: "Bioregulatory and psychosocial forces collude to push sleep onset later, yet schools are timed to begin earlier across adolescence, and sleep time is compressed as a consequence."

Right away, when researchers looked at the effects of early start times, they found they were easily linked to sleep deprivation. In 1998, Carskadon studied the sleep of ninth graders who started school at 8:25 a.m. and again in tenth graders who started at 7:20 a.m. in Rhode Island. She found the groups went to bed at the same time, with the 7:20 a.m. kids waking much earlier and suffering significant sleep deprivation. At the time, she wrote: "Imposition of an early school start time may require unrealistic—if not unattainable—bedtimes to provide adequate time for sleeping."

Certain school districts became aware of this information and made changes. In Minnesota, the state's medical association recommended to all Minnesota superintendents that high schools start later, making the point that "there remains an erroneous societal concept that sleep is negotiable, rather than a biologic imperative." First Edina, Minnesota, then the Minneapolis Public Schools heeded the advice. Minneapolis shifted the start times of its seven high schools, starting with the 1997–1998 school year. High school moved from a 7:15 a.m. start time and 1:45 p.m. dismissal to an 8:40 a.m. start time and 3:20 p.m. dismissal. The change would have a profound effect on some twelve thousand students.

Opponents to the change argued that if school started later, the kids would just stay up later and wouldn't actually get more sleep. This did not happen. Researcher Kyla Wahlstrom at the University of Minnesota tracked the Minneapolis students and found that after the schedule change, they were going to bed at the same time, on average, similar to the Rhode Island students, and sleeping one hour more in the morning.

The researchers also found striking differences in how the kids felt. When the start time was set at 8:40 a.m., the kids were less likely to report feeling sad or depressed, hopeless about the future, tense, or worrying too much. They were less likely to say they arrived late to class, fell asleep in class, or felt sleepy while taking a test, reading, or studying. In a focus group, the kids reported the general sentiment that they couldn't imagine returning to the earlier start time. One described the feeling of the early start time as "I can hear stuff. But I'm a lot more detached and tired. I can't concentrate." They expressed that when it came to bedtime, they couldn't fall asleep before 11:00 p.m. or midnight even if they tried. In focus groups, the teachers nearly unanimously agreed that students were more alert and not sleeping at their desks. Principals said they were dealing with fewer disciplinary issues. The front offices were less congested in the morning, as fewer students were tardy. School counselors and nurses said that fewer students came to them with peer conflict issues or difficulty with their parents. Suburban parents almost unanimously supported the change, and parents in urban schools had a more mixed response, with some citing the difficulties associated with work and transportation changes. And yet, tellingly, parents across the board reported that their kids were "easier to live with" and that they had more connection with their kids because, instead of rushing and having confrontations in the morning, they were having real conversations.

The effects didn't fade. Even after four years, the kids with the later time continued to get an hour more of sleep every night of the school week.

With funding from the CDC, Wahlstrom expanded the Minneapolis study to include eight high schools in Minnesota, Colorado, and Jackson Hole, Wyoming, all of which had shifted start times from 7:30 a.m. to between 8:00 and 8:55 a.m. Overall, an 8:30 a.m. start time allowed the majority of the students to sleep at least eight hours a night. Across all the districts studied, the kids who slept more than eight hours a night were more likely to say they were in good overall health, and less likely to report feeling depressed or using caffeine or other substances like alcohol, tobacco, and other drugs. There was also a statistically significant increase in GPAs for the core subjects, and absenteeism and tardiness was reduced.

In Jackson Hole, after the start time was moved from 7:35 a.m. to 8:55 a.m., the number of car crashes for high-school-age drivers dropped by a whopping 70 percent (whereas the rate stayed the same for other age groups during the same period). Fairfax, Virginia, also saw a significant decline in adolescent car crashes after moving the high school bell from 7:20 a.m. to 8:10 a.m. Mahtomedi, Minnesota, saw a 60 percent reduction in crashes for teen drivers after the high school start time was shifted thirty minutes. The same pattern was found in Chesapeake, Virginia, where high schools start at 8:40 a.m. and 8:45 a.m., in comparison to neighboring Virginia Beach, where high schools start at 7:20 a.m. and 7:25 a.m. Data from the Virginia DMV on crashes in which drivers were sixteen to eighteen years old, occurring between Monday and Friday, revealed that the kids in Virginia Beach were involved in 19.2 percent more crashes. A follow-up study replicated these findings with two other Virginia school districts, finding the high school with the earlier start time

---

SLEEPLESS AND DRIVING

Motor vehicle crashes account for 1 million deaths annually, worldwide. An adult who sleeps six to seven hours a night is twice as likely to be involved in a crash than someone sleeping eight hours or more, and sleeping less than five hours increases the risk four to five times. Distracted driving, which is common for all ages, is likely to multiply the effects of sleeplessness. Driving simulator studies indicate that sleep restriction leads to levels of driving impairment similar to those seen in illegal blood alcohol levels.

had more teen crashes and more run-off-the-road accidents, which are often related to falling asleep at the wheel. The issue of accidents is particularly critical, because sixteen- to twenty-year-olds have the highest injury rates from motor vehicle crashes. According to the National Highway Traffic Safety Administration, fifteen- to twenty-year-olds make up only 6 percent of licensed drivers, but are involved in almost 20 percent of motor-vehicle-related fatalities in the U.S.

With our understanding of adolescent sleep needs—and the pile of data on student health and safety—we can clearly see that it would be wise for high schools to end the practice of early start times. There are no two ways about it. If you're a high school principal, a school board member, a superintendent or similar, the only student-centered answer is to shift high school start times to 8:30 a.m. or later. The logistical issues (which we will discuss shortly) will never outweigh the mental health and safety consequences to teenagers. As a parent, the next time you attend a town hall or PTA meeting on student mental health, if your high school starts earlier than 8:30 a.m., raise your hand and ask when your

PARENTS AND TEENS ON SLEEP SCHEDULES BEFORE AND DURING THE PANDEMIC

I have to say, school starting at 9:00 a.m. just feels right.

School starting at 8:30 is sooo much better. It's like a revelation. How did we do this before?

Once we got on the distance-learning schedule, my daughter was in heaven. Six a.m. wake-ups for her to get to school were brutal. For us, even 8:30 a.m. versus 8:00 a.m. would be life-changing.

We switched to a school with a 9:00 a.m.–4:00 p.m. schedule. Life-changing, for sure!

school will be taking this clear and measurable first step—and following the science.

We have to change start times now.

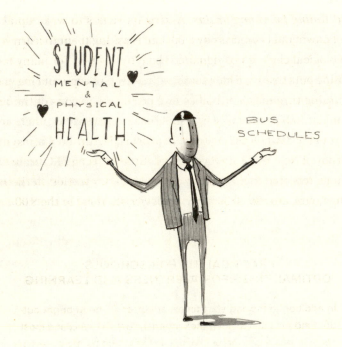

Logistical puzzles should not outweigh student health and safety.

THE MANY WAYS EARLY START TIMES HAMPER LEARNING

The mental health and safety stakes of teen sleep deprivation are certainly reasons to make immediate changes to schedules. But in addition to this, early start times hamper the very thing we want our kids to do in school: learn. If a school's first-period bell rings at 7:45 a.m., it's like pushing students out onto a sea of learning, in a leaky boat. Immediately, they are at a disadvantage.

There are a few reasons that early start times get in the way of learning:

Bad timing for young brains. Asking teenagers to wake up at the crack of dawn and be in class by 8:00 a.m. is asking them to learn when their biological clock is not signaling them to be alert. For many teens, early rising puts them in a half-zombie state—with sleep-inducing chemicals surging through their bodies and prefrontal regions of the brain operating at half capacity. This would be akin to waking adults up at 4:00 a.m. every day and asking them to attend a lecture on photosynthesis. A study of New York City high school students using EEG brain wave recordings reported highest brain alertness and retention in the mid-morning hours, around 10:30 a.m., and lower alertness in the 8:00 a.m.–

PRACTICAL TIP FOR SCHOOLS: OPTIMAL TIMES FOR ALERTNESS AND LEARNING

In addition to moving start times, adolescents need bright outdoor morning sun to keep their internal clocks in sync, and most seem to retain information, think creatively, and be more alert in the mid- to late morning. How can we use this to help kids? First, start the day with time outside. This could mean sitting in a circle to check in about the day, beginning with outdoor PE or a walk around the track (in winter coats if needed), or simply playing music and giving kids time to finish work—the key is *outside*. Morning sun (ideally not viewed through a window) alerts the brain's internal clock, improves mood, and helps kids get better sleep at night. Rigorous academic classes and tests should not take place first thing in the morning. Adults are often early risers and "morning types," so we assume teens will do well early in the morning too, but because of the later timing of the internal clock, this is often not the case.

9:00 a.m. hour. For adolescents, the researchers suggest, "mid-morning may be the best time to learn," which makes sense given what we know about the sleep phase delay for adolescents. We want kids to care about their work, to focus, retain, and feel inspired, but we have hamstrung them with unhealthy conditions. A study of Chicago public schools, most of which start by 8:00 a.m., found that kids do worse in math if they have math first period, or English if they have English first period.

Mental powers are depleted. Early start times simply do not allow kids enough time to sleep, and we know this impairs learning. For example, in a study of adolescents who attend top high schools in Singapore, researchers restricted sleep to five hours per night for one week (if that seems extreme, it's not—many teens find themselves sleeping this little), and found that the kids experienced lower levels of attention, memory, executive function, and positive mood. Not only that, the effect remained even after two nights of recovery sleep, showing how sleeping in on the weekend isn't a fail-safe solution. This dulled thinking and feeling is likely to happen as the higher powers of the prefrontal cortex shut down during sleep deprivation and energy is diverted to the basic functions we need to survive. Yes, teens can walk around, talk, and move their bodies, but the sophisticated brain powers we want them to use operate at partial capacity when they are sleep deprived. Kids who find classes "boring" and take a long time to finish their homework are often flabbergasted when they realize that with regular good sleep, those lectures suddenly seem interesting and homework gets done more efficiently.

Not surprisingly, studies have found associations between sleep and grades. Students who get average grades of B's and above sleep significantly more than those who get C's and below. Remember from chapter 3 that a teen who sleeps for seven hours and is forced awake with an early alarm is missing two hours of REM-rich sleep. REM, or dream sleep, is necessary for emotional processing and mental health. It's also key to memory formation, insight, and creativity. In other words, it's key for school.

In an experiment in an Israeli middle school, a group of students started school at 8:30 a.m. instead of at 7:30 a.m. like their peers, and at the end of each week, the groups took tests that measured their attention and accuracy. The later-start group slept an hour more than their early-start peers, performed significantly better on tests of attention, made fewer errors, and had a quicker reaction time.

Children of color and children from families with lower incomes are at particular risk for poor sleep health. A recent study of elementary school children in historically disinvested neighborhoods found that the kids who had indications of lower sleep were more likely to struggle with behavior issues and academic achievement.

Social jet lag. Another reason that early start times hamstring students is social jet lag. The earlier the start time, the more out of sync the day's schedule is with the natural clock of adolescents. The more severe the sleep deprivation is during the week, the greater the pressure to catch up on sleep on the weekends. Imagine two high school students who have the same workload but different school start times. As we've seen from the research, bedtimes tend to stay the same regardless of start times, so in this case we'll assume both kids go to sleep at 11:00 p.m. and wake at the time needed for school. The calculation for total weekday sleep deprivation assumes nine hours of nightly sleep needs.

STUDENT A: 7:45 A.M. START TIME
Weekday wake time: 6:15 a.m.
Weekday bedtime: 11:00 p.m.
Total weekday sleep deprivation: 8.75 hours

STUDENT B: 8:45 A.M. START TIME
Weekday wake time: 7:15 a.m.
Weekday bedtime: 11:00 p.m.
Total weekday sleep deprivation: 3.75 hours

By the end of the week, student A is missing 8.75 hours of sleep, whereas student B is missing 3.75 hours. (Not bad, student B.) Student A might feel the need to sleep extra on the weekends, let's say until 10:00 a.m. on Saturday and Sunday morning. If we assume a bedtime of midnight on the weekend, that's ten hours per night. This will feel good, but as we saw in chapter 3, this social jet lag means that the internal clock struggles to orient, as the cues of sunlight, eating, behavioral patterns, and social interactions are now severely altered for the weekend. The teen has changed time zones by almost four hours, as if flying from Alaska to New York. Student B has a good option to approach the weekend: sleep in just one hour more each morning, filling up on two good nights of sleep and keeping the internal clock on track and regulated.

Indeed, a recent *JAMA Pediatrics* study tracked high school students' sleep with actigraphs (watch-sized devices that track sleep and activity periods) and found the kids with the earlier start times slept less during the week and more on the weekends—suggesting more social jet lag. Mary Carskadon found that Rhode Island high school students who slept less during the week and had a greater delay in sleep on the weekend had worse grades, along with greater daytime sleepiness and depressive mood.

Let's go wild here and dream up the most teen-centered schedules. What if school schedules were truly synced to the adolescent biological rhythms? A high school in England took this a step further and set the schedule around what they assessed would be the optimal learning time for most teenagers—moving the start time from 8:50 a.m. to 10:00 a.m. (with the option of earlier drop-off one hour before school if parents wished). Sure enough, student illnesses dropped by 50 percent. The later time allowed adolescents to get sufficient sleep, reduced their stress levels, and reduced their social jet lag—all of which are known to support healthy immune function. In New Zealand, a high school made the innovative change to move the start time to 10:30 a.m., but just for students in their last year, when sleep deprivation is known to become acute. Now, that's thinking outside the box.

✧

LEVELING UNEQUAL PLAYING FIELDS THROUGH SLEEP

Unhealthy start times appear to also perpetuate inequities in education, and healthy start times are a policy that helps address these inequities. For example, students who ride the bus are more drastically impacted by an early start time, because bus routes require picking students up much earlier than driving to school. Kids who live closer to their schools, are driven to school by a parent, or have their own car can sleep later. In fact, every minute of commute time to school has been shown to confer 1.3 minutes of lost sleep for students. Researchers at the University of Washington saw that after high school start times shifted later, the high school that saw a significant boost in attendance was the school in which 88 percent were "economically disadvantaged students."

The Brookings Institution, in a report on policies to improve education, concluded that moving start times later is a change to support disadvantaged students. Their analysis found that the earliest high school start times hurt kids from families with lower incomes—to a degree on par with having an ineffective teacher. They note that reading and math scores go up when start times are moved later, but that "disadvantaged students benefited the most, with effects roughly twice as large."

Early rising is accentuated for kids who rely on public and school transportation. And surveys of high schools have found that those in which more families were labeled as "well-off to affluent" were more likely to have healthy start times. If we know that more sleep creates a healthier mental and physical foundation for kids, then we recognize that healthy start times are an obvious way to support all students by taking care of their basic needs. In the same way every family should have access to clean air, water, food, and health care, every student should have a reasonable school schedule that allows them healthy sleep.

It's not hard to see why the American Academy of Pediatrics issued a statement in 2014 recommending that middle and high schools start no earlier than 8:30 a.m., noting that insufficient sleep in adolescents is "an important public health issue that significantly affects the health and safety, as well as the academic success, of our nation's middle and high school students." Healthy start times for teens have also been recommended by the American Academy of Sleep Medicine and the Centers for Disease Control and Prevention, among others.

In 2015, Seattle Public Schools became one of the largest districts in the country to require a healthy start time for teenagers, beginning with the 2016–2017 year. All the city's public high schools and most middle schools were shifted to start at 8:45 a.m. The school board vice president called it a "great win for our students that will unleash a torrent of public schools shifting to bell times that make sense for students."

Researchers at the University of Washington studied the Seattle kids and found they got more sleep, and tardiness and absences went down. They also tracked kids' performance in one of their core classes, biology, before and after the change. The group who started later scored 4.5 percent higher, which researchers and teachers pointed out could be the difference between a B and an A. In interviews about the change, the biology teachers noted that with a 7:50 a.m. start time, the students were yawning and had a hard time focusing or having discussions, and that after the change the kids were better able to engage in "deeper thought and scientific discourse." Absences and tardiness went down (as noted earlier, particularly for the high school whose neighborhood had a lower average household income).

TEENS TAKE SLEEP INTO THEIR OWN HANDS

Jilly Dos Santos was a high school student in Columbia, Missouri. When she heard, in 2013, that her high school was considering moving their 7:50 a.m. start time to 7:20 a.m. to solve busing issues, she took action. She created a Facebook group and a petition, contacted the organization Start School Later, and filled a school board meeting with dissenting teens. One high schooler told the board, "I am already active in too many clubs for my own good. I will not be working at my best. I simply will not be there. I ask you from the bottom of my heart, please do not make me take Calculus 3 at 7:30 a.m." In the end, the board voted against the change. Not only that, Dos Santos's movement created further support for healthy start times and Missouri's Columbia Public Schools voted to move the high school start times to 8:55 a.m. *The New York Times* wrote an article about her action as a teen advocate for healthy practices.

In 2019, California became the first state to regulate high school start times with the passage of SB 328, which requires middle schools to start at 8:00 a.m. or later and high schools at 8:30 a.m. or later. Before the change, a survey of traditional California high schools in large school districts found that only 5 percent of the sample started at the hour recommended by the AAP. Roughly half were starting in the 7:00 a.m. hour, and some started as early as 7:15 a.m. in Westside, Los Angeles, where Heather lives. The Santa Monica and Culver City school districts, along with various independent schools, have already made the change to 8:30 a.m.—a move that became especially clear for supporting students on the heels of the pandemic. Things are looking good for her local high school moving from 7:50 a.m. to 8:30 a.m. as well—which is extra important, as kids come from all over the city and often drive on the perilous Pacific Coast Highway.

WHY THE RESISTANCE?

The health and safety arguments for reasonable start times have histori-cally been neglected. The power of the status quo, fear of change, and perceived concerns over budgets, sports schedules, and other logistical issues have stymied progress.

One of the sources of resistance to changing school schedules is the notion that the district will need more buses and bus drivers to enable fewer delivery tiers. Many districts have found cost-neutral approaches to making the change, while others have decided to invest in a solution that includes more buses and a higher cost. Some have saved money or time. In Fairfax, the district considered several different options (includ-ing a cost-neutral one), before settling on a plan that added 27 new buses to a fleet of 1,600, for a cost of roughly $5 million (in a transportation budget well over $100 million). To put this in context, the total budget for the school district was $2.5 billion.

Another issue in moving schedules has been the influence of sports and the concern that shifting dismissal times later may bump up against early-afternoon activities, meaning practices could be moved or short-ened. Parents worry that kids may get home later and older kids may not be as available to take care of their younger siblings in the afternoons. Grappling with these changes means creative problem-solving among parents, schools, and coaches. Some schools have found that existing practice and game schedules still work or need only minor adjustments. Others have worked to coordinate regional changes in start times for sports so that schools in the same league all have similar schedules. Add-ing lighting to outdoor fields for later practices in seasons when the sun sets early, making before-and-after care available at school, and strategi-cally rearranging school periods to accommodate student athletes are other creative solutions to these logistical challenges. Schools that have made the change have found ways to do so that are cost-effective, maintain vibrant sports and extracurricular activities, and provide appropriate start times for kindergarten to twelfth grade.

The impact on sports was a concern when Minneapolis high schools made the start time change. A few coaches whose teams had long practices and travel times did complain, but participation in sports and other after-school activities overall remained the same. Generally, coaches and activity leaders were pleased with the change and noticed the kids were more mentally alert at the end of the day. In Wilton, Connecticut, considered a "sports town," the Wilton Sports Council was a tough opponent to the change. They insisted that any change in start times would lead to the expulsion of Wilton teams from the athletic conference, a price too high to pay for any other possible benefit. In the end, though, after implementing the change, Wilton High School had one of its best athletic seasons, and participation in extracurricular programs actually went up. The only problems were for students who had to be pulled out of class early for away games and for students who participated in more than one sport, although this full schedule would be difficult with any school start time. For the most part, research shows that when start times move later, involvement in activities does not go down.

Plenty of athletic directors and coaches have noted the benefit to high school athletes. For example, when St. George's School, a college prep boarding and day school that had forty-eight sports teams, moved their start time to 8:30 a.m., the director of athletics and head football coach said, "We have found it one of the best things our school has ever done." In fact, athletic coaches should be first in line to support healthy start times, as we know that sleep boosts athletic performance and lowers the risk of injury. When the college swimming and basketball teams carved out ten hours for sleeping, their reaction times and performance improved significantly. The Boston Red Sox built a "sleep room" at Fenway Park to allow players to sleep, thus giving them a competitive edge. Sleep increases growth hormone and testosterone, and leads to quick decision-making, precision, and better endurance. Sleep consultants now work with the NBA, MLB, Olympic teams, and other such groups—so why aren't we protecting and optimizing high school players' sleep? When high-performing athletes and medalists understand and tout the value of sleep, but student athletes are stuck with six hours because their school starts at 7:30 a.m., something is not right. Our high school athletes should also get the benefit of good sleep—injuries will go down, and performance will go up.

The organization SLEEP in Fairfax compared two real students and their respective schedules at an early-starting versus a late-starting school. The sports practice times turned out not to be that disparate from one another. For various reasons, many practices were already starting more than an hour after the school dismissal time. See the comparison on page 125 and decide which seems more humane to you.

Here's a testimonial from Loudoun mom Jane: "We love the late start schedule. Clearly there is a great deal of research that supports this approach for high school kids since they need so much more sleep at this age. We never have to argue in the morning about getting up like most parents and teens in other localities."

Changes that are good for mental and physical health also often come with long-term financial benefits, which is why it's no surprise that several groups have shown the economic benefit to later start times. RAND Corporation researchers calculated the boost of higher academic performance (for example, one hour of sleep gained, on average, increases the probability of high school graduation by 13.3 percent and college attendance by 9.6 percent) and reduced car crash rates and concluded that after two years of moving all U.S. high school start times to 8:30 a.m. or later, the economic boost would be $8.6 billion. After a decade, that would rise to $83 billion in benefit, and after fifteen years, $140 billion. They noted in their report that this is likely to be a conservative estimate, as it did not include the uplifting effects of a reduction in mental health issues and a lower incidence of physical ailments like obesity and future heart disease. The Brookings Institution estimated the benefits to costs

Loudoun County high schools start at 9:00 a.m.
Fairfax County high schools start at 7:20–7:30 a.m.
How does the schedule work for students?

SEAN'S SCHEDULE IN LOUDOUN		MARIA'S SCHEDULE IN FAIRFAX
Sleeping	5:00 a.m.	Sleeping
Sleeping	5:30 a.m.	Alarm rings
Sleeping	6:25 a.m.	Bus stop
Sleeping	7:00 a.m.	Arrives at school
Alarm rings	7:30 a.m.	Calculus class
Bus stop	8:25 a.m.	Calculus class
Calculus class	9:00 a.m.	AP Spanish
AP Spanish	10:35 a.m.	Lunch
Lunch	12:12 p.m.	AP Literature
AP Literature	2:05 p.m.	School's out
	3:15 p.m.	Cross-country practice starts
School's out	3:45 p.m.	
Cross-country practice starts	4:00 p.m.	
	5:30 p.m.	Practice ends
Practice ends	6:00 p.m.	
Dinner with family	6:30 p.m.	Dinner with family
Teens with later-morning start times fall asleep at about the same time at night as students who start school earlier in the morning and do sleep longer. The hormone required for sleep peaks later at night in teen brains—typically at about 11:00 p.m.		
Lights out	11:00 p.m.	Lights out
8.5 hours of sleep		6.5 hours of sleep

Source: SLEEP in Fairfax

of moving middle and high school start times later as 9 to 1, pointing out
that school reformers and policy makers often talk about broad changes
like expanding charter schools or implementing more rigorous standards

CREATIVE SOLUTIONS FOR SHIFTING SCHEDULES

Install lights on athletic fields

Make last period of the day a flexible period for students on a sports team that needs daylight hours to practice

In 2021, Garnet Valley, Pennsylvania, high school moved to an 8:35 a.m. start time and kept their dismissal time the same, at 2:35 p.m., but changed the schedule of classes to take advantage of an increase in flexible, "asynchronous" learning for students.

to boost student achievement, but they overlook more "mundane" reforms, like schedules, that could have a big impact at a lower cost.

The idea of changing the status quo around early start times seems to offend and anger people to a surprising degree—in a way that can't quite be explained by costs and sports schedules. Is it something deeper about catering to or coddling teenagers, who we think should toughen up? Is it denial of or anger at the idea that science should inform our basic daily life? When you consider the health and safety of kids and the long-term financial benefits on the one side, and the initial output of funds and logistical headaches required to change schedules on the other, it's so clear which side should win out, so the resistance to change is emotional, not rational. You can see this in the comments on stories describing the latest study of harmful effects from teen sleep deprivation. The reaction from many is "Yes, this makes sense," but some of the comments are surprisingly negative toward teenagers. Kyla Wahlstrom, who studied the Minnesota changes and benefits, noted the resistance to change, even in the face of facts, as being somewhat about politics and leaders in administrative roles not wanting to take risks or being afraid of the backlash. Inaction is the result of this hesitation. "The process of change," she says, "is unsettling to most people."

SHOULD ELEMENTARY SCHOOL STUDENTS TAKE THE EARLY SHIFT?

One of the solutions to the high school start time dilemma has been to rearrange the bus tiers to make the elementary schoolers the ones who start early. Elementary schoolers naturally tend to go to bed early and wake early, so this may make sense. In fact, a recent study of start time changes in the Cherry Creek School District in Denver, Colorado—in which elementary start time was moved an hour earlier, to 8:00 a.m., so that middle and high school could move to 8:50 a.m. and 8:20 a.m.—found that the younger kids' sleep stayed the same, while older kids benefited. How early is *too early* for this age group has yet to be determined. Little kids need their sleep too—in fact, many kids in the younger elementary grades need 11 to 12 hours of nightly sleep, so cutting too far into their sleep time is not good. To illustrate this, let's take an example of a healthy sleep schedule for a kindergartner to second grader, as well as a middle schooler:

Early elementary schooler
Bedtime 7:30 p.m.
Wake time 7:00 a.m.
Sleep needs: 11 to 12 hours per night

Middle schooler
Bedtime: 9:00 p.m.
Wake time: 7:00 a.m.
Sleep needs: 10 hours per night

Moving elementary students earlier so middle and high school students can start later may be a solution—but schools should be cautious about taking this too far and starting little kids before 8:00 a.m., especially if it's a school in which families need to commute distances to get there.

Phyllis Payne saw the resistance for years as she worked on moving school start times in Virginia. After her babysitter described waiting for the high school bus in the dark, another student she knew came down with a case of mononucleosis that would not go away. She was a healthy teen, captain of a sports team, but she just wasn't recovering, and Phyllis remembers thinking, *This poor girl really needs more sleep.* Despite the fact that parents, students, pediatricians, and others repeatedly asked for relief from the 7:20 a.m. start time, collected thousands of signatures, formed advocacy groups, and presented clear evidence about the harm being done to the kids, it took almost two decades for the school board to approve the change. As a new mom, when she first became aware of the issue, Phyllis heard that the PTA had already brought it up, and she remembers thinking, *When my daughter gets to high school, this will obviously have been sorted out.* Her daughter had graduated by the time Fairfax High School start times were moved to 8:10 a.m.

ACADEMIC OVERLOAD AND STRESS

At a school board meeting in Greenwich, Connecticut, where moving start times was hotly debated, one of the board members noted: "We're asking if we should change the start time, but I think the real question is how to reduce student stress... Changing the start time is only one part of it. The other part is the amount of homework we have, the amount of AP courses that we take..."

Setting reasonable start times for schools is a high-impact first step. But addressing student overload will also be vital to regaining good sleep. In high schools all around the globe, kids are loading up on classes, enrichment activities, and other work and academic responsibilities, to an often unhealthy extent. The attitude of more is always better creates pressure and stress that make balance and healthy sleep virtually impossible for teenagers. Many teens don't feel they have control over their lives because everything they do is for a future goal, and is determined by parents, teachers, principals, and coaches. Even for high-achieving kids who have perfect grades and are on every team and in every club, not feeling in control of their lives (doing everything for a future, external reward) can lead to anxiety and depression. Educational reform is outside the scope of this book, but we cannot meaningfully improve teenagers' happiness, peace of mind, self-care, and sleep without talking about ways that academic life could work in harmony with these goals rather than against them.

Take the issue of homework—which has a significant impact on adolescent sleep. The research consensus is that homework in elementary school has no academic benefit and leads to more family conflict and negative attitudes toward school, and yet almost every single elementary school assigns homework, starting in kindergarten. Heather asks teachers at her young daughter's school about this, and one of the most surprising answers they give is that parents *ask* for more homework. They worry their child will fall behind if it's not given. High school homework has limited use, and can be harmful when it takes many hours every evening, raises stress, draws away from family time and downtime, and reduces sleep. A survey of high-performing high schools in California showed that kids were spending an average of more than three hours per night on homework (many reported much more than this). More than half the kids said homework was a primary source of stress, and the researchers saw a connection between students' stress and physical impacts—migraines, ulcers and other stomach problems, sleep deprivation and exhaustion, and weight loss. Many kids expressed feeling like it was pointless busywork, they didn't enjoy it, and that it detracted from hobbies. A mom of three teenagers told us she started a petition in her high-achieving New Jersey district because her junior in high school sometimes had seven hours of homework a night (we had to clarify she really meant seven, and she did), depending on tests and project schedules. She had a heart-to-heart with her son about AP classes and shared with him her concerns about the overload, and he decided to take fewer APs than his peers. (He's on his way to medical school, which we mention as proof that ambition does not have to translate into unhealthy high school overload.)

PRACTICAL TIP FOR SCHOOLS: RETHINK AND CAP HOMEWORK

We often consider lots of homework as a given, must-do part of teaching. But what if homework was flexible, student-driven, and limited, serving to connect material learned in class to the real world? In middle and high school, is there a way to rethink your homework policy to value quality over quantity? Instead of assigning twenty math problems that repeat what was taught in class, can you assign five and tell kids to hang out with family and friends (and get a good night's sleep)? Can their homework be to listen to a podcast on how engineers used math to design the latest spacecraft?

From a child development and brain perspective, the changes schools can make to reduce student stress are the same ones we'd recommend to protect healthy sleep: increasing choice in students' learning (giving students a sense of control in order to increase a feeling of agency and reduce anxiety and depression) and focusing more on helping kids figure out what makes them tick rather than memorizing and meeting standards. Many school curriculums and classrooms are set up around older ideas about teaching: short, frantic classes chosen by adults, bells that ring (too loud and too early), and punishments handed out for stepping out of line. This leads to less intellectual stimulation, less student happiness, and less sleep.

Even the CEO of the College Board wrote in *The Atlantic*:

The typical application for college today has eight to ten spaces for students' activities outside of class, and parents and students have become convinced that the more spaces filled, the better. Long lists cultivate busy mediocrity rather than sustained excellence... MIT recently revised its application to include only four spaces for extracurricular activities, and admissions officials there are evaluating whether they can move to three. Brilliantly, the school also removed the space for students to put any activities from ninth grade on their application. From MIT's point of view, ninth grade is a safe harbor—a year to change your mind, to try different things without regard to your track record.

Interestingly, when we ask parents what they want most for their kids, they almost never give us answers like "I want him to get into the best-ranked college" or "I want her to win swimming competitions." They answer with "I want him to be happy in life," "I want her to feel good about herself," "I wish for him to be a kind person and help others." The message many kids get, though, is that the highest GPA, the most AP classes, and a laundry list of enrichment activities and volunteer hours equal success. It's what therapist Madeline Levine calls a "mass delusion" that can lead to extremely high stress levels for some kids.

Julie: I have this recurring daymare (nightmare when awake) where I ruminate on the messages, like focus on your GPA, the more APs the better, choose activities that will look good on your college applications, etc., that my son got as a high schooler. As a young adult now, he talks about those pressures and time suckers he experienced in high school, and I tell him how bad I feel about it. But it's hard to imagine what it would have been like for him to buck the system in that way. It wasn't only the messages I was sending as a parent; he was surrounded by the very same messages at school, among his peers, in his extended family, and in the world at large. It's not a small thing to contemplate. If I could go back, I would have this conversation with my son then, when he was in the midst of hours of senseless rote memorization and AP study into the early hours of the morning, after three to four hours of lacrosse practice each day. At least then, we could have acknowledged to each other what a big dilemma this was and seen our way clear to taking at least some small, concrete steps to correct his incredibly unbalanced life. He needed not only quite a bit more sleep, he also needed more time just to be a person, a teen, a kid who needed mental space to contemplate all the major existential questions that arise at this age. Having these conversations with families we work with, while they are in the midst of it all, is healing, both to them and to me.

WHAT ABOUT YOUNG ADULTS IN THE WORKPLACE?

We work with young adults whose work schedules also lead to severe sleep deprivation. Many young people work multiple jobs, often totaling sixty to eighty hours a week to stay afloat financially with the high cost of living in today's world. And there are all sorts of careers, from firefighting to investment banking, where the hours worked can easily top a hundred per week.

With schedules like these, getting enough sleep to be healthy and feel good is mathematically impossible. Forget about time to exercise, explore an outside interest, spend time with loved ones, or just relax and have a little fun. What's really sad about these crazy work hours is that businesses could increase the amount and quality of output while saving money simply by reducing work hours. When workers are well rested and their lives are balanced, their performance and inherent value at the workplace skyrockets. Change is slow to come in workplaces like these. It can be linked to the idea that newbies need to suffer and show their mettle, a sort of rite of passage. The irony is, when this is taken too far, the business suffers as well.

SPORTS JUST FOR THE FUN OF IT TOO

Youth sports have become a multibillion-dollar industry: private coaches, high fees for club teams, travel expenses. Kids specialize in sports early, spend many hours a day practicing and many hours on the road competing (at a big cost). Having a genuine desire to make this a central part of family life is great, but some families also tell us it leads to burnout and life imbalance, or that they're doing it for college applications. Indeed, 70 percent of kids stop playing organized sports by age thirteen.

Sports shouldn't be just for elite athletes. The point is to practice, exercise, and benefit from the joy of the game. Some teens will tell us, "Oh, I don't play baseball" or "I'm not a basketball player." But games are games, and adults do not have to organize them. Join the rec league or the YMCA, or just go shoot some baskets, kick a ball on the soccer field, or throw a football with your friends. On your own!

In Korea, academic competition makes healthy sleep impossible. After school ends, many kids go to private tutoring institutions to continue studying and learning, often returning home at 10:00 p.m., where they continue studying. One survey of Korean students found that half are in additional classes until midnight during the week, and the majority attend tutoring lessons on the weekends and during school vacations. The severe sleep deprivation of Korean high schoolers—which has been measured at 4.9 hours per night in some places—is a high price to pay here, especially when we consider Korea's elevated suicide rate. Research indicates that Korean kids who slept less than seven hours per night were one and a half times as likely to contemplate suicide as those who slept more than seven hours.

Is there a better way to educate kids without toxic levels of stress and reduced sleep? In Finland, kids start school at a later age (play is emphasized), take fewer classes at a time, and go deeper into those courses, stay with the same teacher for the long term so they develop a relationship, start school at closer to 9:00 a.m., and have few standardized tests. The focus is on deep, complex thinking rather than rote memorization. A study of homework around the world found fifteen-year-olds in Finland spending under three hours per week on homework, yet they outperform the U.S. in every academic measure. Finland fares exceptionally well when stacked against the highest-ranking countries, including Asian countries. A glance at UNICEF's measures of child well-being around the world tells us that European countries dominate the highest end of the rankings. The Netherlands, Sweden, Denmark, Finland, Spain, Norway, and Germany rank high in overall subjective well-being and happiness, education, health, and other measures that affect the quality of kids' lives. The U.S. and the UK rank at the bottom.

WHAT CAN YOU DO AT HOME?

Choose schools with healthy practices. You may have a choice when it comes to schools, in which case you could choose a school that has a healthy start time of 8:30 a.m. or later (and is close to home, if possible), has significant outside time and exercise, has a homework limit policy, does not encourage too many AP courses, has nontraditional course options, allows students choices, and seems to appreciate that adolescents need downtime, playtime, and family time too. A parent recently told us that her son's high school carved out a protected one-hour lunch break in which parents were not allowed to schedule tutors or cram in another enrichment class or sports lesson—the break was a real break.

    Choose to limit time spent on homework. Ask teachers how much time the student should be spending and communicate with them about that goal versus the reality of how much time the student actually spends. Explore with your teen what will happen if they choose going to bed on time over finishing homework. Will the world come crashing down? Will it motivate them to use their time more efficiently in the future, rather than being forced to stay up until crazy late hours? Letting an assignment slide to get to bed on time might mean a dip in grades in the short term, but cumulatively over time those teens will be more academically successful.

Rethink commitments. Think about the activities and responsibilities you have on your plate. Which ones do you need (for example, a job) or enjoy (a team or hobby), and can you let go of something else to enable you to enjoy a less frantic pace? We find many kids and parents are happier when they choose one or two activities instead of trying to keep up with what they perceive everyone else is doing (social media heightens the feeling we need to be somewhere all the time).

Understand how sleep boosts efficiency. This is an amazing fact about sleep: when you sleep well, you double your efficiency. If you're a teen running on six or seven hours of sleep, you will often procrastinate and then take many hours to complete your homework. When you sleep eight to ten hours, you are more likely to complete your homework earlier and take less time. You'll be happier with the results too, because you'll think more clearly and creatively. Notice how sleep deprivation feeds inefficiency, which then makes it harder to go to bed on time—this is a cycle that you can break by improving your sleep.

Remember the F-O-N-D family. Your F-O-N-D practices from chapter 4: family rituals, open play, nature, and downtime are important components to reducing stress and overload. One day during a recent break from school (which, due to the pandemic, the kids were doing from home at the time), Heather was supporting her daughter with a school assignment to demonstrate the similarities and differences between the praying mantis and the killer bee. With a twenty-five-minute break in between classes, her daughter started working quickly to get the project

PRACTICAL TIP FOR COACHES:
USE SLEEP TO KEEP A COMPETITIVE EDGE

Sleep improves athletic performance and reduces the risk of injury. The factors that give athletes a competitive edge, like accuracy, reaction time, and speed, are improved by sleep, which is why athletes like Tom Brady and LeBron James take their sleep routines seriously. A study of middle and high school athletes found that the amount they slept was the best predictor of injury.

Kids who are driven sometimes can't resist showing up and performing at the highest level, no matter what time or how long practices last. But as adults in charge of kids' well-being, we have to be the ones to model healthy behaviors. Consider reasonable limits on practices and times that aren't too early or late. The good news is that sleep improves skill learning, so practices are more efficient if kids are well slept. Talk to your athletes about how sleep benefits their game, how much sleep they need (9 hours is ideal) and how to improve sleep, based on the habits in chapter 6.

done. "You know what?" Heather asked. "Would you rather skip the next class and keep working on this so you're not rushed?" They decided that, yes, that made more sense. Her daughter spent a long time cutting, gluing, painting, and diligently wrapping sticks with pipe cleaners to make model figures of the insects. Focusing on one project for a longer time made the animal information stick in her daughter's mind more than rushing to the next period would have.

As a parent, high school teacher, guidance counselor, school principal, administrator, or coach, we can all make a difference in putting balance, sleep, and well-being at the forefront for teens. Find like-minded parents and teens and start a group to foster change at your school. Join conversations about reorienting college admissions priorities, limiting the AP classes allowed at your school, creating a less hectic academic schedule, supporting public health campaigns to make it clear that electronics in the bedroom are harmful, and setting healthy school start times. Which piece of the puzzle are you involved in, and how can you make changes—now?

PRACTICAL TAKEAWAYS FOR SLEEP-FORWARD SCHOOLS AND TEAMS

- Move middle and high school start times to 8:30 a.m. or later.
- Begin the day with outdoor time as weather permits.
- In the classroom, leave windows open and shades up in the morning.
- Schedule rigorous academic classes and tests no earlier than 9:00 a.m.
- Teach sleep health alongside other health curriculums like nutrition.
- Try not to schedule practices, clubs, team meetings, and other enrichment before school, and end them by 7:00 or 8:00 p.m.
- Consider after-school homework clubs, and have enrichments and sports take place at school, to cut down on car travel time and to be more friendly to working families. If a child can come home from school at 4:00 or 5:00 p.m. with homework, sports, art, or dance complete, they can have downtime and family time.
- Ensure that you have a clear cell phone policy, one that keeps kids from engaging on their phones during school hours, including during lunch and free periods. Real social interactions during school hours help kids feel connected to one another (remember "Vitamin C," page 87).
- If you have a short school day, consider making these late-start instead of early dismissal days.
- Limit total daily homework assignments. Elementary schools can do away with homework completely, or consider doing so until fourth or fifth grade. See if high school teachers can coordinate

more, so a math test and a massive paper do not land in the same week. Or say, "Here's the homework assignment. Show me how much you can do in forty minutes. No judgment—I truly want to know how you're doing, and what's realistic."

- Create a Zzz's Room at school in which students can sign up for a forty-five-minute time to safely sleep during the school day or between school and practice.

PART II

NAVIGATING THE STORM: PRACTICAL TOOLS

6

The Five Habits of Happy Sleepers

There's nothing more important than optimal sleep.
That's the best way for your body to physically and
emotionally recover. If you can get nine hours, that's amazing.
Sometimes I even get ten hours of sleep.

—LeBron James

We are built to sleep.

Sleep is programmed deep in the human brain, and the instinct to sleep is strong. The undeniable fact is that our bodies crave sleep. Sleep is not something we can force or train ourselves to do. In fact, have you ever tried to "make" yourself sleep? You can't. Sleep is an organic drive. We breathe, we eat, and we sleep without needing to learn how. Sleep is a natural ability we're born with, and like all living things on earth, we already have the instructions.

So why does good sleep feel so elusive and difficult? How could we be in the midst of a public health crisis over something that is a basic, natural human ability?

The answer is that even though sleep is natural, we modern humans actively interrupt and abuse our own sleep so severely that we've lost touch with its power. Artificial lights, electronic media, bright lights, around-the-clock entertainment and news, ever-growing workloads and anxieties, unhealthy activity and school schedules, and more—all suppress the natural biological programming of our sleep. Sleep is there, waiting under the surface, but we are disconnected from the cues and chemical signals of this finely tuned system.

For adolescents, the assault on sleep is much more severe than it is for other age groups (and that's saying a lot). This assault is also unique in *how* it attacks from multiple sides in this particular phase of life. The rest of us do not experience the sleep predicament teenagers do; their struggle to sleep well is different and uniquely challenging. Teenage biology, mixed together with omnipresent screens and social media, academic overload, and early school start times—the perfect storm developing from all directions.

In this chapter, we're going to teach you the practices your teens (and you) can adopt to return their bodies to natural patterns of healthy sleep. Now that we understand how the circadian clock works, how teenagers experience a unique delay in this clock and how they are prone to an even *further* delay from light and mental stimulation, we will translate this knowledge into actionable steps. The steps are what we call the Five Habits of Happy Sleepers. Practicing the five habits will lead to an earlier bedtime, an easier time falling asleep, and longer, better-quality sleep through the night. The results are reduced social jet lag, brighter mood, improved focus and learning, healthier skin and muscles, a boosted immune system, and protection from chronic disease.

Before we learn the five habits, we're going to explain two guiding principles. We teach these principles so that instead of just blindly dabbling at a list of tips, you know the underlying mechanisms. This way, you can adapt the five habits to your own life and circumstances. None of us is perfect or will precisely adhere to every habit every time, but if you understand the "how" behind them, you have the knowledge to make the smartest changes for your family and can feel in control of the outcome.

Let's briefly touch on the two guiding principles first. Then, as you read the five habits, you'll see how all aspects of the habits build and support these two concepts and lead to improved sleep. The two guiding principles help explain why and how sleep functions in the human body. The five habits are actionable steps you can start practicing today.

Principle 1: Paleo-sleep—syncing the circadian rhythms. Sleep is indeed natural, but modern life is anything but. Sleeping well in many ways involves taking inspiration from early humans, because sleep goes back to such an early stage in human evolution, it is built on the idea we still live under the moon and stars. Without artificial light, humans naturally went to sleep and woke up more closely in sync with sunset and sunrise and could adapt their sleeping patterns to the seasons, the length of the day, and other forces of nature. (Don't worry, we're not going to recommend going to bed at 6:00 p.m., but we are going to recommend a distinct wind-down that simulates the setting sun, and five to ten minutes of sunlight in the morning—along with other steps to harness this natural power.) Early humans' timing and sleep chemistry were more closely tied to nature. Artificial light has manipulated our timing in the wrong direction and shortened our sleep, but it's in our control to manipulate it right back.

Remember the camping studies from chapter 3, in which young adults had earlier melatonin onset levels and slept long nights when away from artificial lights? And Max, our wide-awake teen, who struggled until he went to sleepaway camp? In both cases, a closer tie to the sun, darkness, and natural fluctuations in temperature allowed sleep to perform at its best. In our modern lives, 24/7 lights and temperature-controlled environments keep us disconnected from these cues—it's no wonder so many people struggle to sleep.

Sure, we can't camp all year long, but now that we understand the underlying mechanism of sleep, we can bring this knowledge into our daily lives and routines. This concept is what we call paleo-sleep, or sleeping in ways more closely resembling preindustrial humans. And paleo-sleep is particularly useful to help adolescents, because as we've seen, they are more susceptible to delayed sleep than younger kids and adults. The five habits will help teenagers manage their light exposure and timing in order to reduce this delay, and will promote falling asleep earlier and faster, sleeping longer, and feeling more alert during the day. Again, we don't expect teenagers to go to bed at sunset (or even as early as their parents, in many cases), but if we understand the way sleep is naturally built to work, we can more closely sync our circadian rhythms, and the benefit to our teens is enormous.

Principle 2: The sleep bubble—creating the framework for sleep. One of the reasons we struggle with sleep is that we think of it as starting when we get into bed and ending when the alarm goes off. We go, go, go, and then try to jam our sleep into tight quarters, only to start over and do it again the next day. But this is not how sleep works. Sleep begins long before, and ends a good bit after, we hit the pillow. The stage is set one to two hours before our bedtimes, as chemicals rise to prepare us for sleep. During the night, our brains are ready to wake in case of danger, so we must feel safe and resolved in order to sleep well. In the morning, our

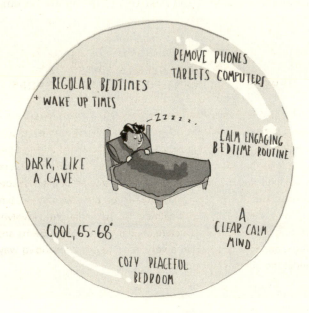

chemistry gradually shifts into alert and productive. These before, during, and after sleep processes are coded in our DNA, and they are tied to the natural cycles of the gradually setting and rising sun, temperature, and other forces of nature.

To harness this wind-down, deep sleep, and "go" morning cycle, we will teach you about a concept we call the "sleep bubble." The sleep bubble takes into account not just the actual night of high-quality sleep you'd like to have, but everything you need before and after sleep in order to make that possible. The prelude to sleep, the quiet peace during sleep, and the mental and physical precedent your day starts with—all are enveloped in the sleep bubble.

As we know from chapter 5, too-early school start times are a way of life for a lot of students. While we work to change that, going to bed earlier is the only possible way for teens to reclaim crucial sleep hours. The name of the game is helping teens set healthy bedtimes and experience more ease in falling asleep. (For many, once they're asleep, jackhammering in the middle of the bedroom won't wake them.) The bubble becomes essen-

---

HEALTHY SLEEP HABITS
VERSUS TREATMENT FOR A SLEEP DISORDER

Sleep disorders like insomnia often require more structured and supervised treatment, like cognitive behavioral therapy. If your teen continues to struggle, lying awake in bed for a long time, after following the recommendations in this chapter for several weeks, it's important to talk to your pediatrician or a sleep specialist about this. In addition to working on the environment, timing, and routines, clinical treatment for insomnia often involves helping adolescents restructure or change thought patterns and associations with sleep in a very specific and prescribed way, under the guidance of a doctor.

tial, because sleep is not something teens can all of a sudden force them-selves to do one night by climbing into bed early and trying really hard. If we think of it this way, it ends in them lying awake feeling frustrated. The sleep bubble is created through all of the five habits—especially by estab-lishing a wind-down time, keeping to a bedtime that is as regular as pos-sible, clearing the room of "sleep stealers," and starting the day with a morning routine. All of these habits will help teens fall asleep earlier and easier and will lead to higher-quality sleep throughout the night.

THE FIVE HABITS OF HAPPY SLEEPERS

The five habits (*SLEEP*) adjust your existing behaviors and routines to be better in sync with your body's natural sleep rhythms, to make falling asleep easier, and to improve the duration and quality of your sleep. The five habits are:

1. S—Set your sleep times.
2. L—Lay out your three routines.
3. E—Extract your sleep stealers (aka "unhelpful sleep associations").
4. E—Eliminate light and make your bedroom a cave.
5. P—Practice a sleep-friendly daytime.

The five habits work together, so the more of these elements you change and improve on, the better your results will be. When you inten-tionally set up your bubble with these five habits, you won't need tricks, trackers, gimmicks, or gadgets to sleep well. Your sleep will self-regulate. You'll experience a greater ease in falling asleep, along with longer and higher-quality sleep. When you enter into your sleep bubble each eve-ning, you'll feel less stressed and in harmony with your body's natural rhythms, which will feed back into a cycle of better sleep.

HABIT #1: SET YOUR SLEEP TIMES

Remember from chapter 3 that you have a timekeeper in your brain. Because of this, having a regular bedtime and wake-up time makes falling and staying asleep a lot easier, and also sets the stage for our highest level of functioning during waking hours. Our outlook, mood, ability to concentrate and learn, decision-making, and creativity improve immensely. A recent study of young adults found that, as expected, more sleep was linked to more positive mood, but more interesting was the finding that the *regularity* of sleep patterns was just as impactful as the amount of sleep they got.

The internal clock is always tracking light, food, activity, and social cues in order to keep our body's systems in sync. What time we fall asleep, wake up, see sunlight, eat, talk to our friends, look at our phones, play sports, and wind down, is logged by the internal clock. If all these cues and behaviors (especially the ones that relate to sleeping, waking, sunlight, and eating) happen at the same time each day, the twenty-four-hour clock learns this timing, begins to anticipate what's next, and helps us by sending the right chemical signals at the right time of day. If you wake at 7:00 a.m. and get sunlight within an hour or two, specialized cells in your eyes detect the light and the signal travels along the optic nerve to the brain's master clock to say: *This is the morning time.* Your brain logs this time and kicks off a cascade of hormonal signals that make you more alert (and also help you fall asleep at bedtime) in the days that follow. If you create a dark environment at home and fall asleep at roughly the same time every night, your internal clock learns this timing and schedules a boost in melatonin production leading up to that time, making it much easier to fall asleep in the nights that follow. The regularity of your sleeping and waking times increases the strength of your chemical signals of alertness and drowsiness.

On the other hand, when you move your sleep and wake times

around, you confuse the internal clock and weaken the signals. Staying up way past your bedtime can cause your brain to worry that something abnormal is happening and lead to a more anxious state. This is your caveperson brain mechanism trying to help you stay alert. It believes you must be awake so late for a reason: perhaps you are on the run or in danger. Melatonin is suppressed and stress hormones rise to help you out. In this way, staying up late and changing sleep times makes it even harder for you to fall asleep when you finally do get into bed. You are out of sync with your body's rhythms, overtired but strangely activated. Since twenty-four-hour clocks exist in organs and cells throughout the body, it's no surprise that we feel better and healthier with regular timing.

MELATONIN SUPPLEMENTS AND OTHER SLEEP AIDS?

There is a place for sleep aids, under the guidance of a trusted doctor, and you should talk to your pediatrician or a sleep specialist about this as a temporary treatment, if indicated. However, for most people, the body's natural chemistry is strong and adjusting your sleep habits will lead your own melatonin to increase in strength. If your teen is really struggling with sleep, talk to her doctor about whether it's best to first get a clear picture of her *natural* ability to sleep, using the strategies in this chapter, before considering seeing a sleep specialist, who may suggest a sleep aid or medication as part of a structured plan.

Now for the reality check: regular timing is one of the most challenging habits for adolescents, to say the least. For one, early school start times force many teens to wake up when their brains are biologically timed to be asleep, so they are forced into an external schedule that is out of sync with their internal schedule (which produces social jet lag). Then, many teens will go into full vampire mode on non-school nights—

hanging out with friends or playing a video game until the wee hours (remember, technology is more than happy to prey on a teen's delayed sleep clock). The morning after staying up late, a teen is in deep sleep when his parents get up to make breakfast, grab the paper, and start the day. He's having full, elaborate REM sleep dreams when his little sister starts her soccer game at 9:00 a.m. If he finally emerges at 11:00 a.m., he's completed a full night's sleep, but now his internal clock will not allow him to fall asleep anywhere close to his regular bedtime that night, and the jet lag cycle continues.

Working within the confines of the school schedule we currently have, we may not get to perfect timing, but improvement is the name of the game. Improving your sleep timing is within your reach, and remember, even thirty minutes of change make a difference. Every step you take toward improving your sleep timing will make you feel happier, healthier, and more productive.

Bedtime, wake time, and the dilemma of sleeping in

FORMULAS FOR YOUR BEDTIME AND WAKE TIME

In middle school, we recommend calculating backward from school day wake-up time by a minimum of nine hours and ideally ten.

Middle school

Bedtime 9–10 hours before wake time

BEDTIME	WAKE TIME
9:00–10:00 p.m.	7:00 a.m.
8:30–9:30 p.m.	6:30 a.m.
8:00–9:00 p.m.	6:00 a.m.

We list a range for each bedtime. It's best to pick a specific time within that range.

In high school, calculate back a minimum of eight hours, and ideally nine.

High school

Bedtime 8–9 hours before wake time

BEDTIME	WAKE TIME
10:00–11:00 p.m.	7:00 a.m.
9:30–10:30 p.m.	6:30 a.m.
9:00–10:00 p.m.	6:00 a.m.

Note: If you're in the first two years of high school, challenge yourself to set your bedtime according to the middle school formula. This will largely depend on your school's start time and commute. If you can do this, you will reach the gold standard of health and well-being. You'll feel stronger, faster, brighter, and more alert and productive with nine hours of regular sleep. Your friends and teachers might comment on how sharp and bright-eyed you seem. And just as important, you'll start to bask in the glory of feeling on top of your game.

TURN OFF THE LIGHT WHEN YOU'RE ACTUALLY FEELING SLEEPY

Yes, we want you to get to bed on time, but we also want you to actually be sleepy when you do. When you first start putting a regular bedtime into practice, move your bedtime *gradually*, by ten minutes each night, until you get to your desired new bedtime. It's really helpful to do this so you don't lie in bed and feel frustrated and sleepless.

On bedtime and broccoli

Prioritizing and protecting a regular bedtime is like Sleep 101. A regular bedtime (along with the right routines and other habits) makes the sleepiness hormone melatonin rise and body temperature go down—both of which are key to falling asleep and sleeping deeply. If a regular bedtime sounds boring, hear us out. Yes, going to bed on time sounds like something your mom tells you to do, along with eating your broccoli. But what if your skin glowed, your muscles were stronger, you got taller, you were faster at track, and the world looked brighter? These are the benefits of regularly timed sleep. Not boring after all.

We can't snap our fingers and change school start times or instantly create a high school homework limit (oh, how we wish we had that power). But putting *sleep forward* and creating a regular bedtime is within our grasp.

Hold on a minute, though: you can't necessarily climb into bed tonight at 9:30 p.m. and fall right asleep (although don't let us keep you from your bed if you're tired). Simply getting into bed early can lead to frustration if you haven't practiced the other habits in this chapter at the same time. A regular wake-up time, morning sun, healthy daytime habits, wind-down routines, a dark room, and technology cutoff times are key to making a regular bedtime work. Remember, sleep begins well before you get into bed.

There's no doubt that a regular bedtime for a teen who has to get up early for school is challenging. It is also potentially life changing. Of course, there will be times when your regular bedtime gets delayed for exceptional reasons, like a school project or a late practice, but in these cases, you're staying up past your bedtime rather than not having one at all.

The goal is to hold on to bedtime, with an hour or less variation, even on the weekends and holidays (see below). When kids are in middle school and the beginning of high school, it's reasonable for parents to still have some control or at least input on healthy weekend bedtimes, but as the end of high school or college approaches, parents are gradually losing control over this aspect of daily life. At this point, parents can model good sleep and technology habits, and talk to their teens in a way that increases their self-motivation (see page 225).

Wake time: Greeting the sun and pressing go

When we wake up, see the sun, eat breakfast, and start talking to our family or friends, these actions press go on our internal clock. Melatonin levels go down and the activating chemical cortisol rises. For the rest of the day, our alertness, problem-solving abilities, hunger, activity, and many other functions of the brain and body will be synchronized through this "go" signal. A regular wake time is also directly linked to falling asleep easily at bedtime.

LIGHT THERAPY

Light therapy is used to improve adolescent sleep, in particular when a teen has extremely delayed sleep timing (falling asleep very late and difficulty waking in the morning). Light therapy involves exposing the person to specific wavelengths of light, for a specific duration, at a specific time of day. When light enters the eye, the signal travels along the optic nerve and to the suprachiasmatic nuclei (page 50) to tell the brain it's morning. Bright light exposure is used when teens wake up, and in some cases the timing of this wake-up and exposure is gradually moved earlier and earlier, as the circadian rhythms learn this new time and begin to advance. With consistency, this resets and reinforces a teen's earlier wake-up time and earlier bedtime, and allows the brain to learn this pattern. For most teens, sunlight can achieve this effect. However, if they aren't interested or able to do this in the way prescribed (either because of the climate or because it's not realistic), portable and even wearable light devices can be used instead. Light therapy has the effect of resetting the internal clock and increasing alertness, as well as acting as a possible antidepressant over time.

For adolescents, wake-up time is largely dictated by school. Depending on when school starts, how you travel to school, what morning responsibilities you might have, and how much time you need to get ready, this is how wake-up time is set. If you're waking up in the 7:00 a.m. hour, that's pretty good (although 8:00 a.m. would likely be the most natural). If you have to be awake in the 6:00 a.m. hour and you're awake late at night, this can be very hard. We know plenty of teens who have to be awake in the 5:00 a.m. hour, and this can be dangerous.

A short, enjoyable morning routine and five to ten minutes of morning light will help boost the biological powers of your regular wake-up time.

Resisting the glorious sleep-in

On the weekends and holidays, the temptation is to stay up late and make up for lost sleep by sleeping in, but when we lean into this too much, it exacerbates social jet lag and also makes the transition to Monday morning extra hard. As luxurious as sleeping in on a Saturday morning can feel, if we take it too far, it comes back to steal our sleep later on. On weekends, since very few high school students have gold-standard sleep during the week, the best approach is to split the difference, sleeping in some, but not so much as to confuse the body clock. For most kids in middle and early high school, one hour past their usual wake time is enough to enjoy the benefits of a full night's sleep, without going too far off the weekday schedule. If your teen has an extreme schedule that requires significant sleep deprivation during the week (we can't ignore the reality for some high schoolers with very early classes and mountains of responsibilities), then he might need to sleep one or two hours later on the weekends. When it comes to shifting back into school mode after a weekend or holiday, see if your teen can gradually move bedtime and wake time fifteen minutes earlier a day to get ready.

Keeping wake-up times regular on the weekends and school breaks and getting five to ten minutes of sunlight in the morning are extremely helpful for keeping your brain in sync and falling asleep at bedtime. Over the summer, teens might shift to a "summer schedule" that aligns more closely with their natural body clock. Remember that sleeping in makes it very difficult to fall asleep at bedtime that night, so the cycle continues. We often recommend that teens who struggle to fall asleep at bedtime and need help syncing their sleep-wake clocks have a summer job or camp that requires getting up and being outdoors in the morning. See page 179 for morning light tips, which can help on the weekends as well.

Generally, we do not recommend naps for children between the ages of five and fifteen years old because naps can make it hard to fall asleep at night and can contribute to social jet lag. After age fifteen, if your high school start time is very early and you have team practices and a lot of homework, you may be accumulating so much sleep debt that napping is a helpful coping tool. See more on napping on pages 183–184.

Let's put this together and consider schedules, including weekends:

Middle school
Bedtime 9–10 hours before wake time

BEDTIME	WAKE TIME	BEDTIME (WEEKEND)	WAKE TIME (WEEKEND)
9:00–10:00 p.m.	7:00 a.m.	10:00–11:00 p.m.	8:00–9:00 a.m.
8:00–9:00 p.m.	6:00 a.m.	9:00–10:00 p.m.	7:00–8:00 a.m.

High school
Bedtime 8–9 hours before wake time

BEDTIME	WAKE TIME	BEDTIME (WEEKEND)	WAKE TIME (WEEKEND)
10:00–11:00 p.m.	7:00 a.m.	11:00 p.m.—12:00 a.m.	8:00–9:00 a.m.*
9:00–10:00 p.m.	6:00 a.m.	10:00 p.m.—11:00 p.m.	8:30 a.m.*

If you sleep in later than this on a Saturday, see if you can at least stick to this schedule on Sunday morning—this way, Monday will not be such a shock. Note that we also made 8:30 a.m. wake time for the high schooler who has to wake at 6:00 a.m. on weekdays because 6:00 a.m. is such an early time; we recommend 8:30 a.m. as a way to make up for lost weekday sleep but not get too far off track for the internal clock. This teen could also wake at 9:00 a.m. on Saturday to make up sleep and 8:00 a.m. on Sunday to get ready for Monday morning.

Simple alarm clocks

A good old-fashioned alarm clock is key for each family member and essential to keeping screens out of bedrooms. The best alarms are:

- **Dark (not illuminated) in the night.** This seems like a small detail, but it's not. Light sends signals to the brain that it's time to be awake. Checking the time or feeling distracted by the light and numbers you see in the night is likely to activate the brain. Find a clock that is dark all night.

- **Low tech and quiet.** Your alarm should be simple and quiet, not connected to the internet or other information, and without interesting functions. Go for a minimalist design and function. We like analog clocks with hands (versus digital numbers) because often they're not illuminated and are simpler. Seeing numbers in the night is too much information for your brain and can create anxiety and sleeplessness.

- **Set for wind-down too.** Ideally, choose a clock that can be set for two alarms. You could use one alarm as your cue that it's time to start winding down and putting away devices before bed and the second one for your wake-up time. This way, you'll establish clear external timing cues (no nagging needed), keep screens out of bedrooms, and have a strong tool for training everyone's internal clock.

- **Snooze and lose.** Don't push the snooze button. Snoozing does not gain you quality sleep and can disrupt your sleep patterns; it doesn't help you feel less foggy and disoriented when you get out of bed. It's much better to set your alarm for when you truly have to get out of bed (rather than setting it early to doze repeatedly). If you have a soft spot for the snooze button, put the alarm across the room on a dresser or shelf so you have to get out of bed to turn it off.

Heather's son, who is in middle school, likes to read before turning off his light to go to bed. She got him a sleep-friendly reading light that does not emit blue or white light (which suppresses melatonin and delays sleep). Heather's husband ordered him a timer that has no light (it's specifically made to be simple and boring, with only one function). This allows him to decide how long he will read for (fifteen or thirty minutes, usually) and then know it's time to turn out the light. This way he doesn't need a phone or a clock of any kind to know when it's time for sleep. This solution works especially well for a child who does not use an alarm clock.

Priorities and time management

Excessive homework and lots of activities (and often late practices, games, meetings, jobs, and events) can make healthy sleep schedules mathematically impossible. A high school freshman told us that he decided not to try out for varsity basketball because it was too physically and mentally taxing and time consuming. This was a big decision, but one that ultimately made him really happy. He was into computers and he focused on that (and he went to college for computer science). Sports are beneficial in so many ways—physically, socially, for self-discipline, to develop a skill you have for the rest of your life—but teens cannot do it all. If we don't model and advocate for balance and self-care, they can be pushed to a sleepless and unhealthy state. An energetic eighth grader whose family spent hours on the road traveling for baseball—which they all loved—told us he was slipping in his grades. We suggested he skip the additional strength training he was trying to fit in every evening. Sure enough, he was able to sleep more, which led to him feeling better and being more on top of his homework. (Side note: He hit a two-run homer in the championship game.)

When you have a full schedule, shifting when you do things can make a difference. What is your trickiest or most daunting task—maybe even something you're dreading doing? Move it to the top of your list. This reduces the very understandable procrastination that arises the longer we wait to tackle the more difficult stuff. Remember that good sleep boosts your productivity and efficiency. If you're falling asleep while reading, your head is going cloudy while you're trying to write a paper, or it's taking you days to finish a project you thought you'd be able to do in a night—sleep will help you with this.

HABIT #2: LAY OUT YOUR THREE ROUTINES

The 24-hour sleep bubble timeline

Okay, let's step into our relaxing sleep bubble, starting with wind-down. Remember, we need a prelude to sleep—we can't just burst in at the last minute and have the bubble carry us through the eight to ten hours we need every night (good for you if you're someone who can!). Most of us have to intentionally create our bubble. Creating three routines will help you accomplish this. Two of these routines come before sleep, and one comes after. All support the sleep bubble.

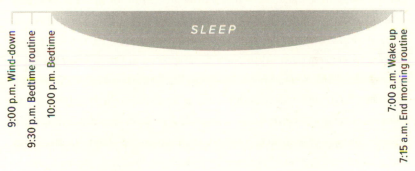

Sleep is supported by the routines before and after it.

By their very nature, routines are predictable and repetitive. They also provide a wonderful cushion of protection around our sleep bubble. Humans of all ages thrive on the predictability of routines, especially when it comes to the sometimes-fragile feelings we can have at bedtime. Routines help us to not think so much and feel calmer as we shift to automatic pilot mode. We feel better when we know what to expect and have the structure to support it.

You have three routines:

1. Wind-down routine (one hour before bedtime)
2. Bedtime routine (fifteen to thirty minutes before bedtime)
3. Morning routine (ten to thirty minutes after waking)

WIND-DOWN ROUTINE (ONE HOUR BEFORE BED)

One hour before bed is what we consider wind-down time. Wind-down time is not a set activity but rather a shift in your focus and surroundings. It's a *relaxed feeling* created by lowering your stress levels, not having big conversations about finances, college plans, or school drama, and turning away from interactive, flow-inducing video games, emails, texts, and social media. Sleep scientist Matthew Walker points out that you wouldn't park your car by driving 60 miles per hour into your garage. This is the idea of wind-down—the prelude, or the slowing down we need for sleep to occur. Wind-down is a time for the mind to focus on more passive (but still pleasurable) activities that help us relax and let go. An important aspect to wind-down time is to *decrease light* in the home. Turn off bright lights and put away phones, tablets, and computers. When you do this, you are adopting your paleo-sleep mentality— simulating sunset and night cues and stepping into your sleep bubble.

The two wind-down factors, *relaxed feeling* and *reducing light*, are simple, but will take time to become a new habit. Both wind-down and bedtime routines engage a Pavlovian response with the regular cues and behaviors we go through before sleep.

The relaxed feeling and reduced light allow us to feel resolved and settled, which protects the sleep bubble. We step out of the way so sleep can take over. Adolescents, who are prone to delayed sleep and whose evening hours are inundated with endless mental stimulation from their phones, computers, homework, and connecting with friends, need this shift to wind-down time even more.

WIND-DOWN DOS	WIND-DOWN DON'TS
Dim lights	Have all the lights on in the house
Say good night/see you tomorrow to friends	Continue texting with friends
Watch a movie on the television	Work on your laptop in bed
Draw in your notebook or write in your journal	Play video games
Read a book you really like	Watch YouTube videos
Change into the new loungewear you picked up during the pandemic	Still be in your school clothes
Walk the dog	Start an exciting project
Finish a baking project	Eat a giant enchilada
Play Boggle with the family	Look at social media
Take a warm shower or bath (helps lower body temperature, which aids falling asleep)	Text your best friends about school drama
Talk about the funny things the dog did that day	Talk about an emotionally charged decision to quit the basketball team
Talk about what you did in robotics class	Start researching how to save for college
Share family stories	Approach your teen about how he should be better at cleaning up
Watch *2001: A Space Odyssey*	Watch *The Conjuring*

Resist the impulse to check one last email or read your texts during wind-down. We see you. Not even one! Really, we mean it. It takes discipline, at first, as does making habit changes like closing and putting away your computer and phone purposefully, in a designated spot, not in your bedroom. Those messages will still be there in the morning, when you can more effectively think about and act on them. If you glance at your phone for just one last look, you are likely to see an interesting, exciting, puzzling, frustrating, or some other emotionally activating piece of information. That last peek also shines light directly into your eyes, sending "time to be awake" signals to your brain. Now you have popped your sleep bubble.

We use wind-down time to great effect with babies and little kids as they absorb the shift to a calmer, slower feeling in the home. Since they have to nap and go to bed earlier than their parents, wind-down prevents their fear of missing out (FOMO) on whatever activity is still going on. They get the feeling that the whole household is going to rest or head to bed. We have them wave *nite-nite* to the living room and kitchen, out the window, and to the pets before being taken into their bedroom to start their routine. Now, as they let their bodies pull them into sleep, they feel settled, resolved, able to let go. Not only is falling asleep easier, but they are much less likely to wake up suddenly and too soon, wondering what they're missing out on. Wind-down time helps with teenager FOMO as well.

BEDTIME ROUTINE (FIFTEEN TO THIRTY MINUTES BEFORE BEDTIME)
Babies and little kids have the grandest bedtime routines. Bath time, singing songs, reading books, cuddles, and all the other thoughtful and sweet rituals that parents come up with and treasure. Typically we see that by middle school parents are becoming looser about routines and kids are putting themselves to bed (often with unhelpful sleep associations). By high school, bedtime routines are often gone completely.

The science and psychology of sleep clearly dictate that we all, no matter our age, sleep better and feel better when we have bedtime routines. Our bodies receive cues to release melatonin and begin to shut our arousal systems down. Our minds receive cues to slow down, say good night to friends and family, put our active thoughts to rest, and let go of the day. The predictability of steps that unfold the same way each evening shifts our routines to our subconscious, which you know from chapter 4 is key to creating a new habit. The steps of a sleep-conducive bedtime routine send signals to our brain that sleep time is near.

A good bedtime routine includes practical steps (charge remaining devices in another room, dim lights, change into pj's, brush teeth, wash face) and enjoyable, relatively passive steps (having a last chat with a family member, journaling or reading a book). If your teen likes to take a warm shower or bath before bed, that will become one of their last steps. Research suggests this can aid in falling asleep.

Examples of bedtime routines:

YOUNG ADOLESCENT

Brush teeth

Change into pajamas

Write in journal

Read a book in bed (sleep-friendly book light)

Last chat with parent, sibling, or caregiver

Lights out

MIDDLE ADOLESCENT

Change into pajamas

Watch an episode of a TV show with family on the couch

Brush teeth

Last chat with parent

Read a book in bed (sleep-friendly book light)

Lights out

OLDER ADOLESCENT

Have a cup of herbal tea and last chat with family

Take a warm shower

Brush teeth

Write in journal

Listen to an audiobook, meditation, or music with a timer set
    to turn off (see page 169 for more on passive distractions)

Lights out

> ## THE LOST ART OF READING A BOOK
>
> Reading for pleasure has been on the decline for some time now. In the late 1970s, 60 percent of twelfth graders said they read a book or magazine almost every day; by 2016, only 16 percent did.

Write down your routine. Clear steps that we write down lead to a feeling of agency and ownership. You can include any silly, sweet, and alluring steps you like. Say good night to pets, plan the breakfast menu, take a hot shower in a dimly lit bathroom, put on a face mask, listen to a podcast, or whatever makes the routine appealing.

MORNING ROUTINE (TEN TO THIRTY MINUTES AFTER WAKING)

In the morning, create some time and mental space in your bubble, which means not jumping up to play a video game, return text messages, or scroll through social media. Just as you did with your bedtime routine, let your mind focus on something simple, interesting, or pleasant, rather than inviting in the complicated issues of news, school, and social life and popping your bubble. Many parents have told us that their kids play video games in the morning on the weekends, and surprise, they wake up extra early! Heather saw this when her kids were in elementary school, so she protected morning time for eating, lounging, playing, reading—anything offline—and it led to her kids miraculously sleeping until the right time in the morning. Try to give yourself ten to thirty minutes of a pleasant and simple routine before you check work and social alerts. This may feel nearly impossible at first, but give it a try. Before you know it, you've created a new habit.

Example of a morning routine:

Splash water on your face
Drink a glass of water with lemon

Take a shower

Put on some waking-up music

Look outside and check the weather

Get dressed

Make and eat breakfast outside for five to ten minutes

(If you need or want to check email and updates, this is a good time
to do it)

Brush teeth and apply sunscreen

Check your backpack, homework, and activity supplies for the day

On the weekend, take the dog for a walk, sit outside and write down what you dreamed about in a journal, shovel snow, or go for a bike ride. All of these expose you to helpful morning light.

HABIT #3: SPOT YOUR SLEEP STEALERS (AKA "UNHELPFUL SLEEP ASSOCIATIONS")

For many of us, especially teens, sleep is delayed and suppressed by what we call unhelpful sleep associations or sleep stealers. These are a sneaky and powerful band of factors that are all too happy to push us to stay awake too late or wake us in the night. Sleep associations are the behaviors and sensory cues in our environment as we are getting very drowsy and falling asleep, such as reading on our phones, talking or texting with our friends until we're very sleepy, the sounds of music or a TV show, the sounds of waves from a sound machine, darkness. (Can you spot which are helpful and which are unhelpful from this list already?) All the things we do, see, and hear right before we fall asleep are our sleep associations. Sleep associations control our sleep to a surprising degree because of the psychological and behavioral patterns they create in our minds. Over time, they become linked to the act of falling asleep and our bodies come to expect them. No matter our age, we all have sleep associations. The problem is that many of us unintentionally create unhelpful ones that make it harder for us to mentally disconnect and fall asleep, suppressing our sleep chemistry and disturbing our sleep during the night.

You can think of your sleep associations as the very last step of your bedtime routine. They include environmental cues like darkness, cool air, the sounds of a fan or nature sounds, the sounds of a podcast or the feeling of the sheets. But they also include the thoughts and feelings you have as you fall asleep. People have told us they imagine a hike in the woods, or floating on the water or on a cloud in the sky (helpful). Others have told us they worry about the future or ruminate about the past (unhelpful). These environmental cues or thought patterns can become sleep associations if they happen repeatedly.

When you spot unhelpful sleep associations and remove them, what comes next is actually surprisingly easy, because helpful sleep associations are simple, logical, and specific to each person. Creating helpful sleep associations is actually the easy part, because sleep is natural. It's removing the unhelpful ones that can be tricky and where your teen (or you) might feel some resistance.

Think about the end of your bedtime routine and what's going on as you fall asleep. Here's how to know if your sleep associations are stealing your sleep.

Sleep stealers/unhelpful sleep associations make it harder for natural sleep to take over and make waking in the night more likely. Unhelpful sleep associations are:

1. **Day signaling/paleo-sleep unfriendly.** Light sends alerting "It's day" signals to our internal clock. Phones, tablets, computers, TVs, and electric lights in our home are sleep suppressing because the light sends signals to the brain that it's not time yet to release melatonin, making falling asleep more difficult; we're just

not sleepy. Remember from chapter 3 that adolescents are already biologically more vulnerable to later bedtimes because of the delayed circadian rhythms and sensitivity to light. Having a string of LED lights in your bedroom or looking at your phone are both sleep stealers. A fifteen-year-old recently told us that during the pandemic, he moved his computer into his bedroom for school, but he recently discovered his computer's mouse was glowing and swirling light and that made it harder for him to fall asleep. A great discovery on his part, and he recognized it as a sleep stealer.

2. **Engaging.** Sleep associations that stimulate our thoughts, interests, and emotions will keep you from sleeping. Anything that makes you feel anxious, angry, sad, curious, excited, scared, or jealous will keep you awake when your body really wants to sleep. Texting, scrolling through social media, playing a video game— all of these keep the mind engaged and delay bedtime, often by hours. These interactive diversions carry us along in a state of flow, finely calibrated by algorithms that tech companies use to keep us occupied and unaware of time passing. Teens who have trouble falling asleep due to negative thought patterns often turn to video games and social media to distract them and help them fall asleep. The problem is that these distractions ultimately delay sleep because they create a state of engagement and flow that makes it hard to stop. See passive distractions on page 169 and the relaxation tools in the appendix.

3. **Externally focused.** Sleep associations that cause us to reach outside ourselves versus letting our natural internal self-soothing ability take over are also sleep stealers. As with engaging sleep associations, the most common examples are falling asleep while

interacting with our electronic devices. If a teen climbs into bed and scrolls through social media, plays a game, watches YouTube, or video chats with a friend, she falls asleep in a state of activation, wondering, worrying, and checking something in the external world. This will make it harder to fall asleep. It can also cause night wakings, because if she falls asleep this way, when she comes into a light sleep during the night she may instinctively reach to check the phone or think about the game, video, or conversation. When externally focused sleep associations are in place, our sleep is delayed, choppy, short, and inadequate, and our delicate sleep bubble has popped.

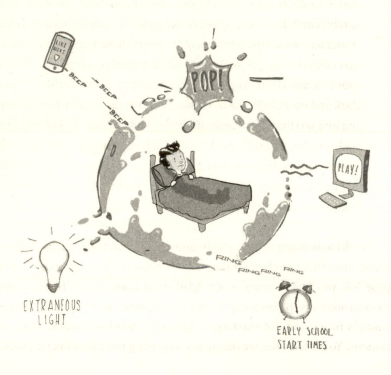

4. **Changes between bedtime and middle of the night.** If light, sounds, scrolling, checking, interacting, and so forth are in place when you fall asleep at bedtime, you're likely to wake in the night because your brain notices something has changed. Numbers 2, 3, and 4 work together, because when we fall asleep in a state of engagement with something external that turns off or changes later in the night, the tug of that unhelpful sleep association is likely to pull us out of sleep. This could be the thought that a text might have come in, a worry about the last thing our friend told us, a new idea about our video game, or the change in sound and light because we had the TV or music on. Waking up this way can give us a jolt of anxiety. It disrupts our sleep and makes it harder to fall back to sleep easily. As part of our natural sleep cycles, we partially wake up about every ninety minutes throughout the night. We rarely remember these episodes because they are so fleeting, but if unhelpful sleep associations are in place, those brief partial wake-ups can become full, wide-eyed awakenings. Imagine a scene in a movie where the protagonist gets lost out in the wilderness. It gets dark and eventually she falls asleep, curled up under a tree, shivering and terrified. Inevitably, in the wee hours, she sits bolt upright, wide awake, instantly back in that activated, frightened state. Of course, this is more extreme than falling asleep directly after playing *Call of Duty* or even after helping a friend sort out a dilemma, but the brain reacts in a similar way.

It's extremely important to spot and remove your sleep stealers. Once you've done this, your helpful sleep associations can emerge. In the list on page 168, you'll see examples of helpful sleep associations. Helpful sleep associations are paleo-sleep friendly (darkness and cool air), boring (sounds funny, but not-exciting is the goal), directed inward, and continuous. You'll see what we mean by comparing the following two lists.

HELPFUL SLEEP ASSOCIATIONS	UNHELPFUL SLEEP ASSOCIATIONS
A dark, cool room	Light
The feel of our blankets, pillows, and body position	Phone in your room, in your hand, or on your pillow as you fall asleep
A quiet room, nature sounds, or a fan	Playing video games
Space in our minds, our own thoughts and imagery	Sending and receiving texts or emails shortly before or while falling asleep
Simple meditation or relaxation breathing	Scrolling through social media or news updates shortly before or while falling asleep
Passive distractions: listening to certain music, podcasts, or audiobooks (if you need this, turn off before falling asleep; see page 169)	Watching YouTube videos or similar
Having your comfy pj's on and climbing into your cozy sheets	Video calling with a friend
	Reading a book on your phone
	Stressful conversations in bed or shortly before falling asleep
	Super-intense, scary, or compelling videos, movies, or television shows playing shortly before or as you fall asleep
	Falling asleep on the couch or other location rather than in bed
	Sounds that change or turn off in the night

Note the sleep associations that apply to you. (Julie likes to use relaxation breathing in a very dark, cool room, using many pillows to get comfortable. Heather turns on a fan and her book light to read, and then she closes her book, plumps up her favorite pillow, and lies on her side, pulling her covers over her ear, just so.)

Helpful sleep associations tell the brain that nothing interesting, worrisome, or engaging is happening. Everything is normal and safe, resolved and settled. We are done for the day. When we do this, the brain is allowed to release the chemicals it needs to induce sleep. Helpful sleep associations are your favorite pillow, the sounds of a fan or rain from a sound machine, your sleep mask, peaceful thoughts, or a sleep meditation. Helpful sleep associations direct your attention to your own self-soothing rather than outward to an external concern or activity and are easily accessible throughout the night. For example, closing your book, plumping up your pillow, getting into your favorite position to sleep, and thinking about something simple for ten minutes. Helpful sleep associations stay the same throughout the night, like darkness or the sound of a fan that continue uninterrupted until morning (versus nodding off with a TV show on).

Teens who feel that their brains are wound up may need a little more help turning off their internal chatter. Let's look at some ways to help them calm their minds, while still keeping only helpful sleep associations.

Passive distractions: Are they sleep stealers?

Listening to music, a guided meditation, or a podcast as you fall asleep seems like a good idea, but these activities can turn into sleep stealers. For most of us, it's best not to do these, but rather to create a wind-down and bedtime routine that end with something like turning on rain sounds and reading a paper book. However, some teens with amped-up minds, who have a lot of difficulty winding down and getting drowsy, can benefit from additional relaxation practices.

First, we recommend trying a mediation or relaxation practice (see the appendix). If further help is needed, then you can consider passive distractions. Passive distractions are something like an audiobook, podcast, or music. The way to know these distractions are helpful is that they are not intense or too engaging, they do not stir feelings and creative inspiration, and they can be listened to in the dark. This is why a teen's favorite music is often not a good choice, but an instrumental track or some laid-back oldies might actually do the trick. Think about the music you listen to when you're going for a run or getting ready to go out. It pumps you up. Now reverse the essence of that completely—this is your passive distraction music. A podcast that drones on about something disconnected from your own life, like the dancing communication of bees, or an audiobook without a suspenseful plot can be very helpful and pull a teenager away from the persistent chatter of thoughts and worries. We've heard a podcast of two people reading the Ikea catalogue, and we've heard others ramble in a calm voice without much of a story line—this is what we mean by boring. A newer option is listening to ASMR (autonomous sensory meridian response) recordings. We don't recommend watching videos in the middle of the night, but the audio tracks of these recordings seem to help some people. As we know from chapter 4, these passive distractions should ideally not come from a smartphone or other device that can open up the texts, social media, and other connections to the wider world. The best practice is to turn these off when you start to feel drowsy.

It can take a little trial and error to find the right passive distraction, but if you're falling asleep in about ten to fifteen minutes, that's a good sign. There is an endless array of podcasts, stories, music, and guided meditations specifically targeted at helping us fall asleep. If your teen is seeking this type of passive distraction, he can experiment until he finds one that fits.

Passive distractions can become the last step of your bedtime routine (habit two) to form a much-needed transitional bridge between your overly engaging activities and falling asleep. The brilliant aspect of this routine tweak is that your passive distractions are pleasurable, something you can look forward to.

If you find your mind is racing as you try to fall asleep, it can help to write things down in a journal or on a whiteboard before your bedtime routine. See the appendix for more meditation and breathing practices that can help you relax. If you wake in the middle of the night, try using your relaxation breathing or meditation. You can also stretch and resettle your body. See more on this in the troubleshooting section at the end of the chapter (pages 185–188).

THE MAGIC OF SLEEPING LIKE A BABY

When we teach parents of babies and toddlers how to change sleep associations, a baby's sleep often improves within three nights. Over and over we see babies go from waking every hour throughout the night to sleeping twelve hours. This happens so quickly in large part because of the power of shifting sleep associations. After about five months of age, babies are very capable of good sleep, but often parents are still feeding, rocking, bouncing, or holding the baby until they're asleep, transferring them into their crib, and ninja-sneaking out of the room—all of which create unhelpful sleep associations. Why would these sweet and well-intentioned tactics be unhelpful? Because the baby goes to sleep with a psychological sense of dependence, seeking external help and assuming the parent will be there all night long. Later in the night, when the baby comes into a partially awake state, they feel confused, incapable, and the parent isn't there anymore. Now they're fully awake. They cry, so the parent goes back in and re-creates the soothing trick. The baby thus does not access their natural ability to self-soothe, and the cycle continues. Our approach shifts to helpful sleep associations, which for a baby or child are anything they do at the moment of falling asleep that is independent and available to them all night: getting into their chosen body position, sucking on fingers or thumbs, holding a lovey or stuffed animal, being alone with their own baby thoughts and sounds. Throughout the night, they feel more confident and turn to these innate abilities automatically, often without having to fully wake up.

It may sound odd, but as teenagers and grown-ups, we are not so different from babies when it comes to sleep. Sure, no one rocks us to sleep (or at least we've never heard that one) or reads us stories and then sneaks out of our room, but we create our own helpful or unhelpful sleep associations that have an equally powerful effect on our sleep.

SIGNALING YOUR PALEO-SLEEP BRAIN
"IT'S OKAY TO SLEEP"

Imagine that you are an early human (because your brain believes you really are). As the sun goes down and you get ready for sleep, you are vulnerable. There are predators, enemies, the elements. Other species have figured out creative ways to solve this dilemma. For example, dolphins sleep with half their brains at a time, while ducks collect in flocks and let the inner members sleep while the outer members keep watch, then rotate, and monkeys sleep in trees. Humans can't do these extraordinary feats, unfortunately. We lose muscle tone when we're in REM sleep, for one, so we'd plummet from a tree if we tried to sleep in its safety.

Still, we have to feel safe in order to sleep. This makes evolutionary sense. As a prehistoric human, if you dropped off into a coma-like state of complete shutdown until morning, you would be in grave danger every night. You'd be attacked, your supplies would be stolen, or you'd freeze from the cold—you wouldn't stand a chance. You need to be able to wake up to solve a problem, go on the run, or defend your family. You sleep, but you are ready. Sure, today there are no lions or a need to migrate in the night to avoid an avalanche, but your brain does not know this. The news, anxieties, questions, fears, bright lights, pings, and alerts of modern life trip the same neurological wires that were put in place to detect these early human dangers. (And let's face it, these days, world events and news stories can actually stack up to feel worse than avalanches and lions.) When bedtime rolls around or when we wake up with a jolt at 3:00 a.m., we find ourselves in an activated state, with our minds racing and our stress hormones rising. Needless to say, it's not easy to fall asleep or fall back to sleep like this. It's not sleep's fault, it's our hardwired, self-protective measures trying to help us.

HABIT #4: ELIMINATE LIGHT AND MAKE
YOUR BEDROOM A CAVE

Going into your cave: dark, cool, quiet

Humans sleep best in a dark, cool, quiet place. We sleep more deeply and wake less often, and the quality of our sleep improves. A dark, cool cave (otherwise known as your bedroom) mimics the darkness and cool temperatures of our natural nighttime and triggers the release of melatonin, so we're working with our paleo-sleep systems.

Controlling the light and temperature in the bedroom are among the simplest yet most influential adjustments we can instantly make. As we know from chapter 3, light and dark are the strongest cues to our internal clocks. As humans, we are not nocturnal creatures—we don't see well in the dark and we aren't built to be active at night (which is why the smartphone is really confusing to our brain). For hundreds of thousands of years, humans saw no light except that of the moon, stars, and fires after sunset. Artificial lights confuse the brain, suppress the release of melatonin, and delay our sleep. Adopting this mentality of cueing your body with well-timed dim light before bed and complete darkness throughout the night (as well as sunlight at the right time in the morning) is a paleo-sleep element that puts you in touch with your body's natural rhythms.

TIPS FOR YOUR SLEEP CAVE

1. **Dim wind-down.** Start dimming the lights one to two hours before bedtime (two is ideal, as melatonin begins to rise well before our bedtime and prepares us to fall asleep). For a teen whose bedtime is 11:00 p.m., this means starting to decrease light in the home around 9:00 p.m. Turn off bright lights in the house, and just use a few lamps. There is some scientific evidence that bright lights coming from above may be more detrimental to sleep because the angle more closely simulates midday sun, whereas lower angle lights on

> ### SLEEP-FRIENDLY READING LIGHTS
> ### AND NIGHT-LIGHTS
>
> The color and intensity of light affects our melatonin production and sleep. Products that are specifically designed to protect sleep and do not interfere with melatonin are sometimes labeled sleep friendly—our families use these as book lights and bedside lamps during wind-down time and bedtime routines. They are often warm-toned and dim. We continue to follow the science and sleep products as they evolve, but it's worth considering a light made specifically to protect sleep. We both use them.

the floor or a table do not. In a perfect world, you'd say good night to your phone and close your computer at this time, but with so much homework to do, teens can find that a tall order. If you have to be on your devices during wind-down time, consider using a light-dimming software that lowers the intensity and changes the color of light on your screens. It's okay to watch TV from a distance, ideally in a room that is not your bedroom, as long as you don't get too sleepy or fall asleep while watching. Experiment with light-blocking glasses. Remember that the dilemma for most teens is the night owl tendency and sensitivity to light. Thus it's actually more important for teenagers and night owls in general to protect wind-down time and have lower lights than it is for adults and morning types, who can more easily fall asleep early for bedtime.

2. **Dark bedroom.** Strings of decorative lights, lamps, and so forth are nice—but turn them all off before you go to sleep. Absolute darkness is the most sleep-conducive. In a sleep consultation with one family, the dad called us the "light detectives." He was spot-on; we are slightly obsessed with darkness because we know how strongly it promotes good sleep. When people describe their rooms as dark

but the curtains don't hang wide or high enough, so the neighbor's floodlights shine in, or digital clocks illuminate the room, or teens have LED lights hanging around their rooms, our radar goes off. You can be a light detective too. Put a sleep-friendly night-light in the bathroom or hallway for anyone who needs to get up in the night. Use blackout shades and curtains in your bedroom. Look out for rays of light around the edges of your windows and do your best to block those as well. This is especially important if you live in an area (like a city) where there's a lot of neighborhood light after the sun sets. If getting your room very dark is too challenging, consider a sleep mask to block the light. Find one that feels comfortable and you'll be surprised at how quickly you get used to it. A sleep mask will help if you share a bedroom, and it's also good to keep one in your suitcase for travel.

3. **Cool night.** The ideal temperature for sleep is between 60 and 68 degrees Fahrenheit/15.5 and 20 degrees Celsius. Sounds chilly to some, but a cooler room helps you fall asleep faster, because as your body's core temperature lowers, this sends signals to the brain and body that it's time to sleep. In fact, your "temperature minimum"—your lowest temperature in a twenty-four-hour day—is in the middle of the night while you're fast asleep. Turn down the thermostat during your wind-down time to help send this signal to your brain. Some research indicates that taking a warm shower or bath, which results in the body's temperature lowering after you get out, one to two hours before bedtime is another way to signal the brain to sleep. Breathing cool air does the trick, while you still feel cozy and comfortable under your covers.

4. **Quiet room.** We sleep best in a quiet room. If you hear a ping or other phone alert, your brain will do its protective duty and pull you awake to check, especially if you're not in a deep sleep. You don't

want any beeps or other sounds to break your continuous sleep and put you in a state of wondering, checking, or anxiety. A fan or a sound machine with nature sounds (not static, but rain or other sounds with variations) is good to use if it helps you. Just make sure it continues all night long, so everything is exactly the same if you wake during the night and it doesn't constitute a changing, unhelpful sleep association. If you share a room, earplugs will also help block noises from snoring, pets, different sleep schedules, and so on.

ORGANIZE YOUR BEDROOM FOR SLEEP

Often a teenager's room is trying to accomplish too much. It's a place to hang out, do schoolwork, store arts and crafts materials and sports equipment, a computer desk and television. The leftover space is for sleeping. This isn't a good setting for sleep because it signals engagement, activity, and interest instead of clearing the mind and creating the simplicity that helps you sleep.

When it comes to a sleep-friendly bedroom, less is more. We understand (because we have teens and young adults, and because we remember the feeling ourselves) that it's important for an adolescent to feel ownership over her bedroom, but there is a way to make the space comfortable for hanging out and also welcome sleep.

Think of creative ways to store and organize your things, and make a space for lounging that is not your bed, if possible. A beanbag chair, floor pillows, a soft rug—anything that gives you the ability to chill in your room but not spend a lot of time sitting on your bed while awake. It can feel natural and comfortable to talk or work on your bed, but this blurs the lines between activity and sleep, making it harder for our brains to shift gears, easily wind down, and be cued by our beds that it's time to sleep. We don't want to dilute the magic of climbing between our cool sheets and resting our heads on our pillows at bedtime by hanging out in our beds for hours at other times. For younger and middle teens, establish this early on, so the habit of doing anything other than sleeping in bed doesn't have a chance to take hold. Especially when kids are younger, homework can be done at the dining room or kitchen table.

Teens claiming their bedroom as a place where they can have some privacy and independence is a normal rite of passage. This became even more common during the pandemic, as teens had nowhere else to go other than their bedrooms to attend online school, do homework, connect with friends, and hang out. If this is the case in your house, see if you can make changes that preserve the sleep-bedroom, or at least sleep-bed, potency. With younger teens, it's reasonable to make this a family agreement (parents should agree not to work or lounge in bed either). As with all of the five habits, parents should have a more direct influence in the early adolescent years. In the later adolescent years, you will shift this responsibility to your teen by appealing to his self-motivation (see page 225) and desire to feel good and be healthy.

Make sure everyone has a workspace that's well-thought-out and comfortable. You may have a corner or nook somewhere in your home where you can create a separate space with a room divider or screen. If you don't have a separate space, that's okay, but do create a space separate from the bed. This can be a desk on the other side of the room and a

PRACTICAL PILLOW PROTOCOL

Adolescent brain researcher Adriana Galván found that teens who say they like their bedding and pillows got better-quality sleep, as measured by actigraphs (wristwatch-like monitors). And those who got better-quality sleep had better brain connectivity—better connections between key brain regions. A teen's affinity for their pillow was a particularly strong correlation, and this effect was true across all socioeconomic lines. Ensuring that teens have comfortable pillows that they like is a low-cost, practical intervention that could have a significant impact on teen sleep. It's also a route through which to address sleep inequities.

comfortable chair for hanging out. If the work/hang space is in the bedroom, when you're starting your wind-down routine, take your devices and computers out of your room and charge them somewhere else during the night. Once, we were working with the parents of a ten-year-old who had a big desktop computer in his room that couldn't be moved back and forth, and for various reasons it wasn't feasible to move it elsewhere. Don't laugh, but we devised a little ritual around "putting the computer to bed" during the wind-down time by turning it off and pulling a light blanket over it. It helped him and his younger brother mentally disconnect from work and games on the computer. They actually started sleeping in later in the morning because, mentally, the lure of the screen was not there.

STEPPING OUT OF YOUR CAVE

When you wake up and see sunlight in the morning, it signals your internal clock that it's day so you can feel alert. Morning sunlight also tells your body when to turn melatonin production back on that evening, making restful sleep more likely at the end of the day. It seems crazy that what we do first thing in the morning can promote falling asleep fifteen hours later, but it does. The internal clock is very attuned and plans way ahead. This means that sun exposure first thing in the morning is key. Read more about this in habit five.

HABIT #5: PRACTICE A SLEEP-FRIENDLY DAYTIME

It sounds strange, but sleeping well is just as much about the *day* as it is about the *night*. The timing of sunlight, as well as the foods we eat and our exercise habits are tracked by our internal clocks. The right daytime practices keep the signals to the clock in sync and support sleep chemistry at night.

Morning light

Getting daily morning sunlight is one of the most powerful habits a teen can practice. As we described in Part 1, seeing sunlight in the morning presses go on the internal clock, which helps activating hormones rise and triggers us to feel alert, energized, and happier during the day, but it also *strongly* contributes to falling asleep more easily at the end of the day. Morning light from the sun works best, so get outside as soon as you can upon waking. Sunlight at noon (while still good for you) is not likely to help your sleep—it should be within an hour or two of your regular wake-up time. On school days, this is best accomplished as a morning routine, or during morning school activities (which is why we recommend schools start the day outside). On the weekend, aim to get outside too. If the sun is shining, five to ten minutes of outside time should do the trick. If you live in an overcast or low-sun region of the world, you may need more time outside to get the same effect. If you can't go outside, open your curtains and window if possible, and face the east, where the sun is rising.

Going back to our paleo-sleep concept, remember that for most of human history we likely rose from sleep close to first light. It was infinitely easier for our early ancestors to be in sync with their natural circadian rhythms than it is in today's world. We have to be very intentional to be in sync because of how modern life keeps us disconnected from these natural cues. People sometimes ask us why they should have blackout curtains in their rooms if we love the cues of morning sun so much. Good question! The answer is that it would be great to use natural morning light if you were also using natural evening darkness. But none of us is really using fully natural darkness (unless you're camping). If morning light was going to be your wake-up cue, you would also want to use natural darkness at sunset. (This is to say, no home lights or screens. Goodbye Netflix and Snapchat.) Otherwise you're harnessing the power of natural light and waking without also harnessing the power of natural darkness and sleep earlier in the night. Your sleep will often be cut short. So, it's best to use light-blocking curtains or shades and to pull them back when you wake up.

Lack of morning light strongly contributes to weekend and holiday social jet lag when teens sleep hours later than on school mornings. Heather gently opens the shades for her adolescent when it's time to wake up, knowing it will make waking up easier (and at a certain time, she lets the dog in, which also does the trick). If your teen gives you permission, you could pop into their room at a certain time to open the curtains or blinds, allowing natural sunlight to help them wake up. Research has shown that morning sunlight on a teen while they're still sleeping can actually help as well. We also like the idea of dawn-simulating lights on morning alarms.

Exercise

Moderate aerobic exercise has been shown to increase slow wave sleep. Aerobic exercise also increases serotonin and endorphins, boosting mood, reducing tension, and enhancing an overall feeling of well-being. Some people are able to exercise in the evening and still fall asleep easily at bedtime. Others do better exercising earlier in the day, due to the activating effects of a rise in endorphins and core body temperature. Teens don't have a lot of flexibility about when they exercise, but still, keep this in mind. If late practices or trips to the gym can be swapped for after-school times, this is more likely to protect sleep.

If you or your teen already have regular exercise in your day, you're all set. If not, know that baby steps will be enough. Walk to and from school or work, park farther away, run up and down the steps at the athletic field, or do a thirty-minute dance or workout class that raises your heart rate and gets your blood pumping.

> **PRACTICAL TIP:**
> **TIMING OF SPORTS PRACTICES**
>
> Having late or very early sports practices and games gets in the way of healthy sleep. This is because exercise late in the evening can make it difficult to fall asleep, and also because the lights kids are exposed to during practice suppress the release of melatonin and delay sleep. Not to mention homework that needs to be completed. As a coach, can you limit late practices, even by ending them thirty minutes earlier? Practices that happen very early in the morning are also harmful to teenagers, whose internal clocks are not set for this. If this seems like a lot of rules around practice times, it is. But teenagers need about nine hours of sleep every night for healthy growth, muscle repair, and mental health. Protecting their sleep increases their ability to learn skills quickly, improves performance, and reduces the risk of injury.

Daytime food affects nighttime sleep

What you eat and when, throughout the day, every day, has a profound impact on your sleep. In a study of healthy adults, eating less fiber, more saturated fat, and more sugar throughout the day was linked with participants getting lighter, less restorative sleep, and with more awakenings throughout the night. Mediterranean diets have been associated with better sleep. Healthy, nutrient-rich foods, eaten on a regular basis, form the building blocks for the chemical environment our bodies require to produce the neurotransmitters that are key to supporting sleep. It makes perfect sense: our bodies and minds work best when balance and harmony prevail across all our systems. It's impossible to separate out exercise, food, or sleep; these foundational pieces all work together and need one another.

Sleep deprivation changes the hormones that regulate our appetite and eating behaviors. The hormone leptin, which signals we're full, is reduced when people are sleep deprived. Ghrelin, which is a hormone that signals hunger, is increased. This means that when we lose sleep, we are more likely to crave and eat unhealthy food.

Sleep-friendly foods: dos and don'ts

DOS	DON'TS
Bedtime snack of cereal, multigrain toast, popcorn, or a banana	Bedtime snack of spicy curry or an enchilada
Herbal tea	A big meal
Flavored sparkling water	Caffeinated soda or coffee after 1:00 p.m.
Sips of water before bed	Energy drinks
	Black or green tea
	Chocolate
	Alcohol
	A jumbo glass of a sugary drink

Caffeine: sleep stealer. When we see teens order a caffeinated soda with dinner or sip an energy drink in the evening and they tell us they have trouble falling asleep, we are far from surprised. The stimulating effects of caffeine can last six hours or longer in our bodies, so having a cutoff time for caffeine is really important. One p.m. is a good time for many teens with an 11:00 p.m. bedtime. Everyone is different, so experiment with your own cutoff time for caffeine. Herbal teas, sparkling water, and filtered water with a squeeze of lemon, orange, or slices of cucumber are good alternatives.

Alcohol: sleep stealer. For you parents, it's understandable to think of alcohol as sleep friendly because it's most often consumed in the evenings and associated with stress relief, letting go of the day, and relaxation. It even tricks us by making us *feel* sleepy at bedtime. But the good news ends there. Drinking alcohol before bedtime makes us more likely to wake up throughout the night. Even if we don't realize this is happening (we feel as though we slept just fine), alcohol suppresses REM sleep and lowers the overall quality of our sleep. We're not saying you should never drink alcohol if you enjoy it. (It's not our intention to be strict and all-or-nothing, but rather to give you the science.) Moderation is the name of the game for most people. But it's important to know that alcohol does affect your sleep quality. This advice is mainly for young adults and parents (although we realize alcohol use is also prevalent among teens).

Bedtime snacks. These are fine, but just as we're winding down, our digestive systems need to do the same, preparing to rest and "hibernate" at night. Eating too much or eating food that is hard to digest puts our digestive systems into overdrive, making it harder to fall asleep and more likely we'll have disrupted sleep during the night.

Smart napping

A nap can easily reduce your sleep drive, which makes it harder to fall asleep at bedtime. Even a ten-minute nap (and even the doze you did not intend to take when you fell asleep on your history textbook) can delay your bedtime significantly, because it releases pressure in the homeostatic sleep drive (chapter 3). This can become a cycle in which you nap, fall asleep too late at bedtime, do not sleep enough at night, and then need a nap the next day, and the cycle continues.

Taking a nap at any time of the day, but especially one in the evening, can delay sleepiness at bedtime. This is good to know, because many teens will crash when they get home from a long day of school, jobs, sports, or other activities, having gotten too little sleep the night before. Crashing like this in the late afternoon, of course, leads to another late bedtime and the need to nap the next day, perpetuating the cycle.

In a perfect world, we'd change policies to limit homework and push high school start times to 9:00 a.m., in which case adolescents would not need to nap. Alas, that is not the reality for most kids. We do find that high schoolers are better off not napping *if* they can instead work on time management, limit pre-bedtime screens, and get to sleep early enough to have 8.5 to nine hours of regular nightly sleep. When this happens, the full attainment of night sleep and no nap keep the body's internal clock in sync and reduce social jet lag.

However, for a high schooler who suffers chronic sleep loss because of excessive homework and early start times, a nap may be necessary and beneficial.

Again, let's talk about perfect worlds: the best time for a teen to nap is in the midafternoon, rather than the evening, with the nap lasting about twenty to thirty minutes (much longer and you go into a deeper stage of sleep that makes you more disoriented and groggy when waking). If we could design a sleep-friendly high school, it would have a Zzz's Room (or an offshoot of the health office), in which students could sign up for a free period to sleep during school hours or in between school and practices. This would allow teens who need to nap *before* the end of a long day the opportunity to do so, rather than coming home and falling asleep while trying to do homework.

❧

PUTTING IT ALL TOGETHER

The Five Habits (*SLEEP*): Set your sleep times, Lay out your three routines, Extract your sleep stealers, Eliminate light and make your bedroom a cave, and Practice sleep-friendly daytime are all key to improving sleep. They work together, so leaving one out will lessen the power of the whole system. If you have a good, relaxing bedtime routine, but you have all the lights on in the house during wind-down, at the last minute you check text messages before bed, you sleep in a lot on the weekend, have a caffeinated drink with dinner, or another piece of the puzzle is missing—the finely calibrated sleep systems are not working in sync. This can lead to frustration and a feeling that it's not working.

Improving *all five habits, for approximately two weeks*, will create a sleep bubble and will allow your natural sleeping powers to emerge and take over. Consistency is key. Imagine us cheering you on as you incorporate the five habits into your daily life.

HERE ARE SOME OF THE MOST COMMON QUESTIONS PARENTS ASK US ABOUT TEEN SLEEP HABITS

The later my teen stays up, the more she seems to forget about sleep altogether. Why isn't she tired enough to just shut down and sleep?

One of the reasons this happens is that the later we stay up, the worse our decision-making becomes. The further a teen goes past her bedtime, the more likely she is to forget her good habits and lose rational decision-making power. So, in addition to how screens and social behaviors delay bedtime, late bedtime begets an even later bedtime as her sense of judgment fades.

Some nights, despite his best intentions, my son just has too much homework to do, for anything resembling wind-down or a healthy bedtime. How do we handle evenings like this?

It's a fact of our modern education system that many teens have an impossible amount of homework. Sadly, it doesn't correlate with improvement in overall learning and achievement. See if there's something he can pare down on. Put away devices, except the ones needed for school, to limit the distractions. Bring up the issue of homework overload at a parent meeting or email the teacher or principal. Consider opting out of certain assignments if they cut too far into sleep. It's normal for teens to feel as though every class and activity is important, because the pressure on them is intense and sadly very future-focused, so it's up to us to send the message that it's more important to follow their interests and take care of their mental and physical health than to win the race everyone else seems to be running. Also remember that good sleep doubles your productivity, so if your teen can get to bed earlier, then he'll be ready to conquer his assignments the next day.

After a full day at school, followed by lacrosse practice, my daughter walks in the door around 6:00 p.m., goes straight to her room, and face-plants onto her bed. She immediately falls into a deep sleep that, no matter how I try, I can't wake her from. She can sleep like this for two to three hours, which pushes her bedtime to some crazy hour like 2:00 to 3:00 a.m. Then she has to wake up at 6:30 a.m. to get to school on time and the cycle repeats. She complains she's so beat and she's ready to drop and says she has to nap. How can I help her?

This pattern is a tough one, as it throws the teen's circadian rhythm into chaos and deprives her of a full night's sleep. The key to helping her is to connect with what she's telling you about how tired she feels. Lead with empathy, listening, and understanding (chapter 8), so you tap into her self-motivation to make changes. The goal is to eliminate the late nap and stick to an earlier bedtime. Give her the info on sleep and athletic performance or the benefits to skin—whatever it is she cares about. She could start skipping the late nap and tough it out until a reasonable bedtime (at least 9:30 to 10:30 p.m. for a 6:30 a.m. wake-up time). Another option is for her to gradually shorten her nap and move her bedtime earlier by ten to fifteen minutes each evening until the nap is eliminated. (This one is tricky because she's in such a deep sleep—she would need to set an alarm and get up herself.) Exposure to bright early-morning light would also help to sync her new, earlier bedtime with her internal clock.

My son tells me that he lies awake at bedtime, sometimes for hours, unable to fall asleep. How can I help him?

Difficulty falling asleep is one of the most common issues for teens. The first thing to do is review the five habits and make sure your son is making adjustments toward protecting his sleep bubble. Early-morning sunlight, not sleeping in more than an extra hour on weekends, and at least one hour of wind-down time before bedtime, in which lights are lowered and screens are limited—all are key. If falling asleep is still challenging, try the relaxation techniques in the appendix, and if this doesn't work, use a passive distraction (page 169). If after two to three weeks of following the five habits and additional relaxation techniques, he still can't fall asleep, it's time to ask for a referral from your doctor to a sleep specialist—preferably one who specializes in cognitive behavioral therapy for insomnia (CBT-i).

My daughter wakes in the night and says she can't fall back to sleep. What should she do?

It's normal for us to wake up in the night. In fact, all of us do, naturally. But when these night wakings go on for more than about fifteen to thirty minutes or so, it's a good idea to make adjustments. If your teen is in bed for only seven or eight hours, then an additional period of being awake in the night can be concerning. First, make sure there are no "sleep stealers" in her room or her bedtime routine. Computers, lights, phones, and other sleep stealers are the number one culprit for night waking. Next, have her choose a relaxation exercise or sleep meditation (see the appendix) to use during the night. After these two steps, if she continues to have a significant amount of time awake in the night, have her try getting out of bed, going into another room, and reading or watching TV (from a distance, not on a handheld device) until she starts to feel sleepy. Then, she can climb back into bed. If after adjusting the five habits and practicing getting out of bed until sleepy, she's still awake in the night, then just as we said above, it's a good idea to seek help from a sleep specialist.

THE TEEN SLEEP CHEAT SHEET

Hi there. We're guessing that a parent, teacher, coach, or maybe another family member asked you to read this little section—or you're reading it on your own. We're so happy that you are! We'll be quick.

Sleep will change your life for the better, no matter who you are. If you're an athlete, sleeping well (8.5 to 10 hours) the night before or the night after practice helps you learn skills and improves your accuracy. More sleep means more growth hormone production, and greater muscle building and repair (so you're less likely to get injured). If you're into robotics, the debate team, video games, creative writing, or anything that requires fast reaction times or creativity, sleep supercharges your prefrontal cortex (that's your smart, focused hub of brainpower). Feeling low, stressed, or overwhelmed? Eight and a half to ten hours of sleep each night balances your stress hormones and boosts your dopamine and serotonin production, which elevates your mood and brings anxiety down. Want to grow taller or have better skin? Yep, more sleep again. (Although something tells us you are beautiful just the way you are.) Have a crush on someone? Well, sleep makes your glass feel half full and brings out all of the amazing unique qualities that make you you.

While your parents may just be talking about mental health, grades, and driving safety (all of which are massively improved by healthy sleep), know that sleep is more than health and safety. It's your secret weapon. Take some time to read this chapter or the summary below and chat about it with a parent, friend, or teacher. Or you could steal this book at night and read it yourself. (But just not too late.) ☺

Here's a breakdown of the five habits that help you get this level of sleep and results. Hint: Notice what word the first letters of each habit spells.

1. Set your sleep times

In middle school, pick a regular bedtime that is nine to ten hours before your regular wake time. In high school, pick a regular bedtime that is eight to nine hours (nine if you're in the first two years of high school) before your regular wake time.

Middle school

Bedtime 9–10 hours before wake time

BEDTIME	WAKE TIME	BEDTIME (WEEKEND)	WAKE TIME (WEEKEND)
9:00–10:00 p.m.	7:00 a.m.	10:00–11:00 p.m.	8:00–9:00 a.m.
8:00–9:00 p.m.	6:00 a.m.	9:00–10:00 p.m.	7:00–8:00 a.m.

High school

Bedtime 8–9 hours before wake time

BEDTIME	WAKE TIME	BEDTIME (WEEKEND)	WAKE TIME (WEEKEND)
10:00–11:00 p.m.	7:00 a.m.	11:00 p.m.—12:00 a.m.	8:00–9:00 a.m.
9:00–10:00 p.m.	6:00 a.m.	10:00 p.m.—11:00 p.m.	8:30 a.m.

Good to know:

Move your bedtime gradually, about fifteen minutes per night.

Do not sleep more than one to two hours later on the weekends unless you are very sleep deprived.

When you wake, get five to thirty minutes of sunlight by going outside.

Use an old-fashioned alarm clock with no illuminated numbers.

Set your alarm for when you really have to get up. Don't hit the snooze button.

2. Lay out your three routines

Limit light and put away devices. Lower your stress and mental activity for about one hour before your bedtime (your *wind-down routine*) so your sleep chemistry can emerge. Otherwise your brain stays alert. This is crucial. *Bedtime routines* signal your brain it's time for sleeping, and the predictability helps trigger drowsiness. *Morning routines* include sunlight, which wakes the brain up and helps you sleep the next night. Examples of your three routines:

Wind-down routine (sixty minutes before bedtime):
Turn off overhead lights in the house, turn on lamps
Take a shower
Put your phone on the charger in the kitchen and your computer in another room
Make a bowl of cereal and watch an episode of TV with family in the living room
(See wind-down dos and don'ts on page 159)

Bedtime routine (fifteen to thirty minutes before bedtime):
EXAMPLE 1
Brush teeth
Change into pajamas
Write in journal
Read a book in bed (sleep-friendly book light)
Last chat with parent, sibling, or caregiver
Lights out

EXAMPLE 2
Take a warm shower
Change into something cozy
Have a cup of herbal tea and last chat with family

Brush teeth

Write in journal

Listen to an audiobook, meditation, or music with a timer set to
turn off

(See page 169 for more on passive distractions)

Lights out

Morning routine:

Splash water on your face

Drink a glass of water with lemon

Take a shower

Put on some waking-up music

Make and eat breakfast outside for five to ten minutes

(If you need or want to check email and updates, this is a good time
to do it)

Check your backpack, homework, and activity supplies for the day

On the weekend, read a book, write down what you dreamed about
in a journal (outside!), take a walk, or go for a bike ride

3. Extract your sleep stealers (aka unhelpful sleep associations)

If your bedtime routine contains a sleep stealer, you will not sleep
as well. Sleep stealers signal your brain to be alert and suppress your
sleep chemistry; they are engaging (like social media or video games)
and directed outward (like texting a friend) rather than inward (like
closing your eyes and thinking about waves in the ocean), or they
change during the night.

Top sleep stealers to remove:

Light in your room

Phone in your room, in your hand, or on your pillow as you fall
asleep

TV or computer in your room

Playing video games

Sending and receiving texts or emails shortly before or while falling asleep

Scrolling through social media or news updates shortly before or while falling asleep

Watching YouTube videos or similar

Video calling with a friend

Stressful conversations in bed or shortly before falling asleep

Super-intense, scary, or compelling videos, movies, or television shows playing shortly before or as you fall asleep

Falling asleep on the couch or other location rather than in bed

Sounds that change or turn off in the night

4. Eliminate light and make your bedroom a cave

We sleep best in dark, cool, boring spaces—which signal to the brain that it's night and there's nothing more to do.

Wind-down:

Turn off overhead home lights, use only lamps

Shut down your computer and charge your phone in another room

Turn the thermostat down to between 60 and 68 degrees

Bedtime:

Turn off all lights, including decorative lights and lamps in your room

Put up blackout shades

Wear a mask if you like it

5. Practice a sleep-friendly daytime

Sleeping well is just as much about the *day* as it is about the *night*.

Get five to thirty minutes of sunlight (even if it's cloudy) before 10:00 a.m. every day, including weekends. The more sun and outdoor time you have in the morning, the better your energy, mood, and sleep. If you like to run, the best time is the morning. If you can, walk or bike to school, keep the shades open in your home or classroom, look at the sky while you're on the bus riding to school, or hand your teacher a copy of this book and ask him to make first period start with outside discussions or a walk around the track—all of this is excellent.

Try not to exercise in the late evening.

Avoid caffeine after 1:00 p.m.

Sleep-friendly foods: dos and don'ts

DOS	DON'TS
Bedtime snack of cereal, multigrain toast, popcorn, or a banana	Bedtime snack of spicy curry or an enchilada
Herbal tea	Caffeinated soda, black or green tea or coffee after 1:00 p.m.
Flavored sparkling water	Energy drinks
Sips of water before bed	Chocolate
	Alcohol
	A jumbo glass of a sugary drink

Naps are a slippery slope. It's best to get eight and a half to ten hours of sleep and not nap; otherwise it's hard to fall asleep at night and creates social jet lag—meaning your body clock is confused. Try not to nap. Try also to get your homework done earlier, put your phone on "Do not disturb" while you're working, and follow the other habits. If you have a job, hours of homework, and practice, along with an early high school start time, then you may need to nap. If so, stick to afternoon (not evening) naps that are twenty to thirty minutes.

7

The Parent Fade

What kind of influence do you have over your adolescent's bedtime and wake time, healthy sleep habits, routines, and so forth? Many parents tell us they feel they've lost all control over this aspect of life. It's true, the nature of your role will change—as it should. It's mind-blowing for us to think about, but since they won't always have us to remind them it's time for bed and tuck them in (lump in our throats as we write this), we do slowly and surely change the part we play. As our adolescents grow, there will be a natural shift from parent-controlled to adolescent-controlled choices, behaviors, and sleep habits.

However, when it comes to sleep, most commonly we see that parents give up their involvement too early. Nearly all our families with ten-year-olds have regular bedtimes and routines, including keeping devices out of the bedrooms. Oh, how things change in just a handful of years: most of our families with sixteen-year-olds tell us they have no idea what time their adolescent goes to bed, and their teen's phone is an appendage they no longer feel they have any control over. With a tween or young adolescent, resist abdicating responsibility for these aspects of life too quickly.

It's still fully reasonable for your young adolescent to have an early, set bedtime and routine, and to have family agreements that keep screens out of the pre-sleep wind-down time and out of the bedroom (see chapters 4 and 6 for more guidance on this). Parents often don't notice how good sleep habits get chipped away, as bedtimes slide later and sleep habits get looser. If you remember deciding on your own bedtime as a teen, also keep in mind that you didn't have the world at your fingertips around the clock. Today's teens can be carried along by technology in an unprecedented way, and the teen brain is especially affected by this mental stimulation and light before bed—chemically suppressing drowsiness and displacing the time they should be sleeping. This means it's extra important to keep family agreements and sleep routines squarely in place through the beginning of high school—remembering that the need for sleep is so beneficial to teens' mental and physical health. Research shows that adolescents go to bed earlier and get more sleep when parents keep up structure around sleep. Parental involvement (that fades gradually) is key to keeping up healthy sleep habits.

For older adolescents, the approach begins to change. You may not have direct control over bedtime. (Heather distinctly remembers her dad announcing "Time for bed!" at 9:30 p.m. throughout high school, which may have been where her appreciation for sleep comes from. Alas, there was less homework and no smartphone or social media to contend with back then.) As older teens take over more decision-making, you can shift from dictating when and how to appeal to their self-motivation to sleep well and feel good. This means giving them information about sleep and helping them see the role of sleep in what matters to them. You could send them an article about sleep, have them read parts of this book, ask them how they feel after a few nights of going to bed on time (remember, teenagers like to feel good too), or point out the role of sleep in sports, health, physical fitness, appearance, creativity, academics—as we know, sleep improves all of it. A dad recently told us that he explained to his son, who plays basketball and wants to be taller, that growth hormone is secreted when we sleep. We thought this was genius. His son likes the idea that as he sleeps, he's supporting as much natural height as possible. In the next chapter, we'll look at sample dialogues for these conversations.

We represent this change over time with a concept called the Parent Fade. Using this tool, you'll see how and when your control over decisions and habits begins to decrease as your adolescent's age and capabilities increase.

THE "ME DO IT!" DRIVE

Your teen was born with a built-in developmental growth factor, imperceptible at first, that steadily and inevitably charges forward. It's not as obvious and trackable as motor skills, language, cognitive advances, and all the other amazing milestones we celebrate, but it's always in the background, driving those other breakthroughs. It's the innate, relentless drive for more and more independence. See how it works:

As soon as your baby can, she rolls, squirms, and eventually crawls away from you. She wants to move and explore every single thing. She desperately wants to become an upright, walking being. She starts expressing strong opinions as young as seven to nine months.

Your toddler incessantly yells, "Me do it!" at every turn and has a meltdown when he isn't quite able to do it or isn't allowed to. He will take risks over and over as the pull of autonomy washes away all reason.

Your preschooler is learning how to do so many new things all by herself. Her curiosity and "why" questions seem endless. The pace is breathtaking. She is very specific about her plans and ideas.

Your grade schooler is seeming more and more like a little person every day. He is exploring interests and hobbies that are separate from yours and loves to play with his friends.

Your preteen is starting to value his friends more and more and to, at times, choose being with them over being with the family. Fitting in and finding identity become the goal. He experiments with differ-ent forms of self-expression.

Your teenager is on her inevitable path to flying the nest. She makes decisions, sometimes big ones, on her own and spends more time with her friend group, separate from the family. She tests rules and limits like never before and may need to push back with strong "Leave me alone" emotions. Becoming autonomous and having more privacy are integral to her crossing the bridge from teenager to adult.

This drive for independence can feel stressful, sad, or like a constant power struggle. After all, your role as a parent all these years has in-cluded managing countless aspects of your child's life. Safety, structure, scheduling, eating, sleeping, screen time—the list goes on and on. At every stage, your role comes into direct conflict with your child's innate tendency to venture out, take risks, resist structure, and generally test limits and boundaries. The intensity increases during the teen years as independence expands to include moving toward an individual identity—a separate self.

Like a projectile hurtling through space, the progression of indepen-dence is built-in and inevitable. As much as we champion our kids' grow-ing abilities and selfhood, the incremental loss over time of their need for us is one of the unspoken sorrows that come with being a parent. As humans, this progression is slower than in any other species, giving us time to savor the early years while also making it harder to let go as they need us less.

Julie: So many of my memories of my son's transitions toward increased independence—leaving preschool, starting kindergarten, middle and high school, first trips away from home, first time walking to school on his own—involve me being an emotional mess, filled with a mix of awe and grief. And living in dread of the inevitable moment when he would leave completely, go to college and wherever life would take him going forward. Like with the contemplation of any great loss, the feeling was that I couldn't possibly survive it, but I did, and when the time came, it felt natural, in a way. What also stands out in my memories is how much less he suffered at these turning points. Saying goodbye easily to his preschool teachers, marching into his kindergarten classroom, relishing school and scouting trips, and generally often appearing as if the next step forward was the most natural thing in the world to him. And it was. This is how we're built.

As parents, when we resist this strong hardwired pull toward independence and try to cling too tightly to our power and control, it can backfire. In our attempt to make decisions for our teens or limit their freedom too much, it either pushes them away ("You don't understand me! I have to go behind your back"), lowers their self-esteem ("Well, my parents don't trust me with this, so I must not be capable"), or paves the way too smoothly for them so they never experience any discomfort.

Kids of all ages are often more capable than we give them credit for. They are innately wired for empathy, learning new skills, problem-solving, and being a significant and contributing member of the group. We have a tendency as parents to overhelp because it's easier and faster to do so (and because it's good to feel needed). This often leaves teenagers with underdeveloped skills in many areas. If we overhelp with practical skills, they may end up not knowing how to cut properly with a knife or fold laundry. If we overhelp with making choices and managing their paths, they may not feel engaged or in control of their own lives.

The "fading" of control is really important, to avoid overhelping your teen. But fading your help as your teen shows you his abilities is different from abruptly letting your teen be in control (which is what we find happens with sleep). In fact, in many realms of life, research and clinical experience tell us that stepping aside completely is not healthy for teens, or for the family as a whole. It may not seem like it when your teen rolls her eyes, answers in one-word mumbles, or does exactly the opposite of what you've asked, but adolescents do need us to be involved, to show curiosity, to impart advice, and to keep communication open. In their book *The Self-Driven Child*, authors William Stixrud and Ned Johnson refer to this as taking on more of a "consultant" role—an important shift in mindset from overhelping to being there as support. They recommend phrases like "You're the expert on you. Nobody really knows you better than you know yourself, because nobody knows what it feels like to be you." The Parent Fade is a delicate dance of conveying trust and sensitively handing the control to your child, who is maturing at a breathtaking pace.

Conflicts and power struggles can make us feel like we're losing our close and loving relationship with our teen. But if we turn this mindset on its head, we can reframe it as a positive natural drive—we can work with it, instead of against it. It's hard to do at times, but let's celebrate what makes teens so extraordinary. Keeping communication going and having an unconditional positive regard toward our kids as their need for autonomy grows are pivotal.

The Parent Fade will help you navigate the dilemmas of handing over control. We will focus specifically on aspects of sleep like bedtime routines and screen agreements, but you can think of the Parent Fade tools in all aspects of teen life.

USING THE PARENT FADE TOOL

The Parent Fade is a simple concept that helps you see your role clearly and avoid underhelping or overhelping. It's a staircase where each flat step represents ways that your teen demonstrates signs of being ready for more responsibility, while the vertical rise to the next step represents you, the parent, increasing your teen's freedom as he shows those signs. The idea is to follow, in a sensitive way, your unique teen's gradual path to independence. It's a flexible evolution that resists either getting stuck in an unnecessary level of control or handing out freedom before it's indicated. It's crucial to know that you're fading only your *control* with this concept, not your connection, curiosity, and interest in your teen. All of those can and should remain high.

The fade starts out with more parental control and less independence and moves toward a full-fledged, autonomous young adult who has taken on more and more responsibility over time. Throughout this progression, teens will ideally have plenty of chances to fail, fall, learn from their mistakes, come up with their own solutions, and make better decisions.

EXAMPLES OF FLAT STEP INDICATORS

Does chores without being reminded

Lets you know where she is when outside the home

Is honest, even when he makes mistakes

Notices the time and starts getting ready for bed without a
   reminder

Honors family agreements like curfews and docking devices in
   the evening

Feels responsible for completing homework

Follows a work-before-play strategy on her own

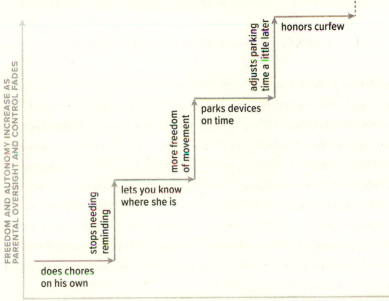

Has found pleasure in activities outside of screens

Shows a level of insight and self-awareness

Has ideas in family meetings

Is open to talking about sleep and health

Tries to figure something out on his own

EXAMPLES OF VERTICAL RISE ACTIONS

Parents stop reminding/nagging about routines and lights-out time

Give teen increased freedom to move around in the world

Parents invite collaborative problem-solving around managing time

Teen is given space to make mistakes

Parents stop doing something for teen that he's capable of doing for himself

Parents give information about sleep, but no longer control sleep
and wake time

Teen becomes responsible for sleep, including bedtime and bedtime
routines

Teen feels a sense of trust from parents

Notice that none of the flat step indicators is age? Age is a clue, but it's not always a definitive marker of the level of responsibility a child is ready for. Adolescents mature at different rates. We don't just want to wake up one day and say, "It's your tenth birthday, here's the latest iPhone!" Automatically handing kids an overwhelming amount of freedom based on how old they are or what their friends are doing can lead to failure and frustration. Instead, flat step indicators are individual behavioral or psychological signs of maturity and capability. If you see your teen shut off their device without your having to mention it or do homework before watching TV, that means it might be time to back off on your reminders so she can start to feel ownership of those choices. On the other hand, if your teen is sneaking his tablet into the room at night (as our friend's son couldn't resist doing), you might have to take a step down the Parent Fade and increase your control over this rule. Put back your clear limits. (You will know when to gradually loosen them again as time goes on.) We know this can be hard, but do not be afraid of pushback.

Even though we're looking for behaviors like honesty, or adherence to family agreements, the goal of the Parent Fade is not that your child does what you say all the time. Teenagers should feel increasing control of their own lives, ideas, and solutions. Your goal is not a mini-me or a child who automatically follows your rules to a T. The Parent Fade looks for more nuanced signs of maturity and allows for collaboration and kids' creative ideas. As it progresses, teenagers get in touch with their self-motivation. Along the way, the fade includes letting your teen fail, make mistakes, and have the experiences she needs to make a better choice the next time—on her own.

YOUNGER ADOLESCENTS

For healthy sleep, middle school kids need a set bedtime, and we recommend doing the math together (see page 154) to find the right one. This also means setting a wind-down time one hour before, including placing devices in a spot away from the bedroom. As the average age for smartphone ownership continues to get younger, saying good night to devices at least one hour before bed is an important practice to establish early on. Remember to share the information about why this is important, because the overall goal is for your child to feel self-motivated. Modeling healthy sleep habits is very powerful too.

Young adolescents often express a desire to have control over their bedrooms, routines, timing, privacy, and so forth—all of which is healthy and normal. This means finding the places they can take ownership, while also knowing the non-negotiables of bedtime and where devices go at what time. We've had many parents tell us that their twelve-year-old has her phone in the bedroom at night; either they don't see it as an issue, or they feel at a loss for how to change it. If it's the former, we would point you back to the research in chapter 4 that clearly links electronics before bed and in the bedroom as delaying and disrupting sleep (and remember, even thirty minutes' more sleep can significantly boost your teen's mental and physical health). If it's a matter of not knowing how to extricate the phone or computer from the bedroom, remember you are the parent, you can set boundaries around such things, and there is a respectful and clear way to do this. See the next chapter for ideas on how to communicate this important aspect of sleep health.

It feels good for your young adolescent to have mastery over parts of his daily schedule, so see where you can pause before automatically doing something for him, correcting him, or telling him what to do. If you don't remind him to put in his retainer before bed, will he? Resist reminding him and see if he does. This is how you'll discover his competency and so will he. A colleague recounted a story of wondering to herself whether her ten-year-old still needed reminding and nudging to brush her teeth. One night she asked her daughter if she had already brushed her teeth, and her daughter said yes, she had. Mom felt her toothbrush: dry. Okay, clearly not ready to fade her involvement in that part of the daily routines!

The young teen years are a good time to teach time management and organization skills. For example, you can show your daughter how to set alerts as prompts, or use an old-fashioned timer or sticky notes. She can begin to use these, or something she chooses, to remember to put her backpack (with homework inside) and soccer cleats, or whatever she needs for the following day, by the front door the evening before. A slightly later alert could signal that it's time to shower and put her phone on the charger at your agreed-upon hour, leaving time afterward for watching a TV show, reading, and having a little pre-bedtime chat. Having timed alerts rather than your reminding (or worse, nagging) is often more effective at nurturing independence. If you do use alerts or alarms, just make sure they're pleasant sounds, not a jarring or negative alarm sound. (Why oh why can't all school bells sound positive, like campus chimes, instead of nightmare-inducing buzzers.) And be sure that, as sleep is approaching, there is a last calm, enjoyable step to look forward to.

While you hold on to structure around screens and bedtime, notice your teen's increasing need for independence. He desperately wants to feel like part of the decision-making process. He needs to know that his voice and opinions are heard and taken into account by you. Invite your teen to learn, brainstorm, and problem-solve around sleep—including talking about the timing, routines, and environment. He will be thrilled to learn that his body and brain, at this life stage, actually are geared to go to bed a little later. You might have a discussion about bedtime during a family meeting where you ask him what time *he* thinks would be good for him to go to bed, given what we know about teens needing about nine hours of nightly sleep. Of course, you're not going to agree to a 1:00 a.m. bedtime, but you might be surprised that your teen makes a reasonable suggestion given the information you share. This is a great moment for your teen to identify what's important to him, and talk about how sleep affects whatever this is. Even attributes like physical appearance and fitness, which are important to adolescents, can be motivators for good sleep.

OLDER ADOLESCENTS

Mid- to late teen brains peak in their hunger for higher-risk experiences and adventures that increase the release of dopamine, the reward neurochemical. As we learned in chapter 2, the reward drive peaks in these years, and good decision-making around time management and bedtimes may be especially challenging for kids around ages fifteen to seventeen because of this peak in reward drive. Formerly rational younger teens can start to make less responsible decisions during this time, as their mental scale weighs more heavily toward rewards than toward possible downsides. Up late at night to keep playing a flow-inducing video game or laugh nonstop with friends? In the moment, these irresistible rewards often outweigh the downsides of losing sleep.

The overall goal is to give teens increasing control—which can feel like a precarious dance. The Parent Fade tool is helpful here because of how different each teen really is in their maturity, need for support and guidance, and number of safe boundaries they need during this pivotal time. If your teen is not making safe choices, you may have to take a step back down the Parent Fade and take over more control, temporarily. It's important not to give up involvement when it comes to health and safety. Just like you wouldn't throw up your hands and let your teen eat fast food every day, you also don't want him staying up late every night and accumulating sleep debt throughout the week and possibly engaging in drowsy driving. Here are some ideas for a sleep-forward mindset in the mid- to late teens:

- Share the information you've learned with your teen in a creative way. Leave this book open on the coffee table or read a section aloud to her, bring it up with her pediatrician, or talk to her coach and suggest a team chat about how sleep improves athletic performance—in other words, you may need a less direct or pressuring way to convey the facts.

- Believe in and appeal to your teen's self-motivation. He likes to feel good, healthy, and happy. Even though he appears to brush them off, the facts do sink in and will contribute to an overall understanding of sleep and shaping of life with sleep as a priority. The problem is that this internal monitor is a work in progress for some teens, and it may take years to develop wise decision-making that will override the temptation for reward. Be patient and don't give up. If you're dismissed by your teen, it's really important that you don't take it personally or become reactive. Keep trying, and keep being an understanding sounding board. Don't forget to use your sense of humor, when appropriate.

- If your teen is chronically sleep deprived, it's reasonable to make better nightly sleep a condition for driving. You would not let your teen drink and drive, so you should not let your teen be sleep deprived and drive. A significant percentage of car crashes are caused by sleep-deprived driving, and adolescents are at the highest risk.

Teens want us to trust them, to listen to them, to give them credit for what they already know. They don't want to be told what to do, or to have things done for them (except they do want you to make their favorite dinner, drive them to meet friends, and regularly wash and fold their laundry). This will manifest as a growing desire for privacy and autonomy. How many of us remember feeling this way as teenagers: "I can make my own decisions, sometimes without even telling you about them!" As a parent, you may find it painful to fathom, but remember how much it meant to you at that age to be trusted and believed in. To resist taking over a situation and acknowledge his need to feel capable and trusted, say empowering things to your teen: "I can see this is tough," "I know you'll figure it out," "Let me know if I can help."

Older teens often express a clear need for privacy, and this is linked to trust. If we trust our kids, we don't need to monitor their every move or intrude on them without asking. If you are seeing the signs that your teen is coping well with more responsibility, as hard as it is, resist the desire to intrude on his privacy. You have already done your job of teaching him right and wrong, ways to stay safe, and good decision-making. If he feels your belief in him, your unconditional positive regard, and your shift to perceiving him as his own person, he will feel closer to you and will be more likely to share and confide in you. Later, when he does have a problem he can't solve on his own, he'll feel safe turning to you for help and advice. Ironically, by backing off gradually, you are shifting to a new role and setting the stage for a deeper connection with him in the future.

8

Empathic and Effective Communication: The ALP Method

I want you to know, I value each of your opinions,
even when you're wrong.
—Ted Lasso

We've explored the perfect storm of factors that collide in the lives of today's teens and compress their sleep to unhealthy levels. We've also learned the habits that protect and improve sleep, harness the power of the internal clock, and bring our bodies into better alignment with our natural sleep systems.

The dilemma for many parents is that, at the end of the day, these changes are tricky to make because they feel at a loss for how to effectively communicate with their teen. They worry they've lost a connection with their child and no longer have any influence or ability to impart advice. They're on eggshells because their adolescent is reactive and will either snap or stop talking, or their teen simply isn't buying this sleep thing—they oppose going to bed earlier, say they're fine, and insist they need to do more homework or hang online with friends.

In this chapter, we'll teach you our three-step method for empathic and effective communication: Attune, Limit-set, Problem-solve (ALP).

We'll also give you plenty of examples to help you through roadblocks. In our practice, we've seen families at every point on the spectrum of family sleep: from families who've lost all semblance of order around screens and bedtime, with every person in their own corner of the house on different devices in the evening and having nonexistent bedtimes, to families with high schoolers who have designated spots to charge devices before bed, no electronics in the bedroom, and regular routines and healthy sleep. What we've learned is that, no matter where you're coming from, communication is key to improving habits and making what seems impossible, possible.

We teach our ALP Method to our psychotherapy clients, first-year parenting groups, teachers, and families because ALP taps into central truths of all human beings. It is key to moving through difficult moments and conflicts, to finding understanding and solutions. The method is explained for babies, toddlers, and little kids in our book *Now Say This*. Here, we will show you how it applies to conversations with adolescents.

ATTUNE > LIMIT-SET > PROBLEM-SOLVE

The ALP Method works for a number of reasons. In the Attune step of ALP, we lead with words or behaviors that convey empathy and understanding. When we attune to another person, we listen actively, without judgment, and are receptive to their point of view. We become aware of their thoughts, feelings, and desires. We see, hear, and take them in; we do everything in our power to understand them, no matter how much we disagree with them or find them illogical. Attuning leads to empathy, which is what we all want and need. In difficult moments, this is the most challenging step and the easiest one to skip. As parents, we often go straight to the rules, our complaints about how our kids aren't listening, or our commands. In doing so, we dismiss their feelings and skip the most valuable part of communication. Empathy is a hardwired and natural human skill, but many of us need to be reminded and guided to practice it by attuning to one another in our daily lives. Often we find that parents are empathic and understanding toward their friends or even other people's kids, but in difficult moments, they forget this simple and powerful approach toward their own children. It's a practice that takes time to become second nature. After the Attune step, setting and holding reasonable Limits and exploring ways to solve the Problem form the second and third steps of ALP.

We've also found over the years that while there's so much beautiful writing and discourse around the practice of empathic, mindful parenting, at the end of the day, parents need a simple and actionable plan. When your toddler is melting down in the grocery store line and you've got fifteen annoyed shoppers behind you, or your teenager breaks her curfew and then lies about where she's been—the parenting books on your bedside table are full of fabulous theories and research, but they may not save you in the moment. ALP is like having the empathic parenting CliffsNotes.

THE ALP METHOD IN ACTION

Attune, Limit-set, and Problem-solve:
Keeping communication open in difficult moments

When we're facing an emotionally challenging moment, we often let our knee-jerk reactions take over. We snap, yell, argue, or throw up our hands in frustration and walk away. The goal of ALP is to stretch ourselves by pausing, listening carefully, and choosing to understand the perspective of the other person, while also holding on to clear limits and thinking of creative solutions. When we take the seemingly easier reactive approach, it often pushes us further apart. When we take the more receptive approach, profound breakthroughs can happen.

Attune (A step) is the first in ALP. In the A step, we let the other person know we understand them and do our best to put ourselves in their shoes. We start by conveying empathy to the other person. When we do this, it connects us and sets the stage for holding limits effectively (L step) and collaborative problem-solving (P step). We are now in this moment together, as teammates with the same goal rather than as adversaries. We let the other person know that we are interested in their point of view, even if it goes against our own, and we're interested in all their feelings, not only the happy, compliant ones. This is essential to moving forward from seemingly stuck places.

The Attune step and Limit-setting step together give you the win-win of parenting. These qualities may seem opposing at first, but they work together and support each other.

WIN		WIN
Warmth	and	High expectations
Empathy	and	Clear limits
Kindness	and	Consistency

Many of the parents we work with operate (with the best of intentions) primarily from one swing of a pendulum. Some parents try very hard to be flexible, kind, and understanding but end up feeling too indulgent and acquiescent. Other parents weigh heavily on unilateral rules and strict expectations. In both cases, parents tell us they feel ineffective, and when their teen pushes back, they end up losing it and yelling, speaking harshly, or reprimanding. ALP gives you a framework for satisfying and balancing *both* of these sides. We see it over and over again in our work with families. Some of us are heavy on the warmth, empathy, and kindness side but cannot hold limits, often wanting to just make our kid happy or choose the path of least friction. Others lean more toward unreasonably high demands and "because I said so" rules. This often results in rebellion or silence and a teen who doesn't feel capable and trusted. Both of these imbalances keep us from a deep and genuine bond. In both swings of the pendulum, trust is compromised.

The win-win concept of ALP will help you understand, collaborate with, and motivate your teen to adopt healthier sleep practices.

THE THREE STEPS OF ALP

Attune—Pause, listen, and lead with empathy. Put yourself in your teen's shoes. Let her know you understand—or are trying to understand—without judgment, her underlying intentions, feelings, desires, and new ways of thinking.

Limit-set—Set and hold reasonable limits consistently. Explain the reason for the limit. If no limit is present, state the reality of the situation.

Problem-solve—Support your teen in coming up with acceptable or more helpful alternatives or solutions.

Step 1: Attune

ALP—Attunement: Becoming aware of and receptive to another person's perspective. Communicating to the other person that you understand, or are curious about, his or her thoughts and feelings.

Teenagers need high levels of empathy and attunement from us. It's important to let them know their feelings and thoughts are okay, that we can handle them and aren't offended, that we're not judging, and that we're curious. This is key to keeping communication open rather than pushing teens away. Adolescence can bring intense feelings, new perspectives on the world, self-awareness, insecurity, a need for experimenting and adventure. During this pivotal time, our kids need us to stretch our capacity to accept and validate their experience by attuning

EXAMINING OUR ASSUMPTIONS ABOUT ADOLESCENTS

How we see adolescents affects how they see themselves, and our relationships. Unfortunately, our society sends us some pretty negative messages about teenagers. Even if we don't think we're affected by the way our culture portrays teens, there may be some subconscious assumptions we hold about them. Examining these assumptions can help us see our kids in a positive, generous light. What if we assumed the very best intentions rather than cynically assuming the worst? If you can be the bigger person and see your teen as good and capable, they will feel this view of themselves reflected back at them and internalize it.

UNHELPFUL	HELPFUL
Teens are self-centered.	Teens have a new level of self-awareness and identity.
She is moody and aloof.	She is probably exhausted.
He answers me in grunts.	He needs me to try a different way of connecting.
Teens are irresponsible.	A teenager's brain is wired for risk-taking and adventure.
I can't get her to talk with me.	She is ready for more freedom or control.
He's lazy and never helps out.	He needs to feel like a capable, significant part of the family.
She seems like she hates me.	It's her way of saying, I need to separate.

(continued)

213

UNHELPFUL	HELPFUL
He only wants to be with friends.	His friends are more important than ever.
Nothing I say makes a difference.	This isn't about me. She needs me to stay and be okay with anger.
When I try to talk, he gets annoyed.	I'm not making him feel seen, heard, felt.
She's moody all the time.	She's suffering, feeling depressed or anxious.

to them. *They need to know that we're interested in knowing the person they are becoming.*

The Attune step is hardest when we're worried about our kids, mad about their behavior, or have hurt feelings ourselves. As parents, we often go straight to stating our point of view, reminding or nagging our kids about the rules, or snapping and yelling. It's in these challenging moments, though, that empathy is needed most. When we shift from our automatic, knee-jerk reactions to a mindful, thoughtful response, it helps our teenagers feel seen as worthy, capable, and valuable people. It raises their self-esteem because they know their experience is valid. We're looking beneath their outward behaviors to the bigger, truer picture.

When it comes to sleep habits, the Attune step is key to softening your teen's defensiveness and to helping him connect the dots himself. You will not always be there to tell him to go to sleep, so instead you'll want to help him feel self-motivated.

There are many ways to convey understanding in the A step. In our practice, we encourage every family to find their own words, body language, and delivery. At first, it really helps to have tools, starter phrases, and examples to help you shift the dynamic. Once you get the hang of it, you will figure out your own way—knowing yourself and your teen. Here are some examples of automatic ways of responding to difficult moments versus attuned responses. Remember that this is just the first of three steps in ALP, so your Limit-setting and Problem-solving steps will come next.

Scenario: Your teen came in past curfew.	
Automatic	You came in past curfew last night—you're grounded!
Attuned	I heard you come in at twelve thirty last night. What was going on?
Scenario: Your teen is still on her phone after you've asked repeatedly for her to put it away.	
Automatic	I've told you a million times, get off your phone!
Attuned	Hey, I know it feels impossible to put it down. Believe me, I feel it myself sometimes.
Scenario: Your twelve-year-old is still playing a video game after you've said it's time to turn it off.	
Automatic	Off, now! Or I'm taking away privileges.
Attuned	You feel like you can't stop, huh? What level are you on? Ah, cool.
Scenario: Your teen says, "All my friends sleep with their phones in their room overnight."	
Automatic	Well, that's too bad for them.
Attuned	I hear you. Grown-ups too! Sounds like you're noticing how common it is to have technology in the bedroom.
Scenario: You have to wake your teen ten times before she gets out of bed.	
Automatic	I'm tired of trying to wake you up in the morning—it's impossible!
Attuned	It's really hard for you to wake up in the morning. I can tell you're so deeply asleep and dreaming. I know the feeling.
Scenario: Your teen has his phone in his room past the agreed-on time.	
Automatic	That's it, hand over the phone. You can have it back in forty-eight hours.
Attuned	I get it, it's hard to find time to hang with your friends when you get home from practice at six and have so much homework to do.
Scenario: Your teen tells you her friend was mean to her.	
Automatic	Oh, I bet you she's just jealous. I don't think you should be friends with her.
Attuned	That must have felt bad. Tell me more.

Scenario: Your young teen is still on his computer late at night.	
Automatic	I give up—I can't control you anymore. Go to bed whenever you want.
Attuned	You've got so much you have to do—and so much you *want* to do—I really see that. It's hard to shut it down.
Scenario: You're trying to ask your teen a question and he yells at you unexpectedly.	
Automatic	Don't yell at me. That's disrespectful! I was just trying to ask you a question!
Attuned	*Pause.* Wow, okay, something's bothering you. I'm here to understand when you're ready.

ATTUNE TOOLS

How you attune depends on your relationship with your child and on the moment. Sometimes it's more body language and tone, with few words. Other times there's more talking involved. You will find your own natural way to convey empathy to your teen over time. Here are some of the best ways (or "tools") to get you started. You can use one or more at a time, depending on the scenario and what feels most natural:

Attune tool #1: Pause, breathe, and say, "Tell me more."

This simple tool will help you resist your impulse to quickly fix, dismiss, or judge your teen's dilemmas, even if you think you already know the answer or are dying to give your opinion. Instead, pause, take a deep breath, and listen carefully. Put your phone facedown, away from you, close your computer, and make eye contact. Nod and just listen, or say, "Ah, okay . . ." or "Tell me more." This expresses your curiosity and invites your teen to share more. Imagine you have no clue or preconceived notion of what your child is going to say, and you're genuinely open to hearing a completely new idea. You will have plenty of opportunities to say what you think, but start with learning more about your teen's point of view. The pause also gives high emotions on both sides a chance to lower in intensity, which can happen in the first minute or two. Time is always our friend in difficult moments.

Attune tool #2: Imagine an iceberg.

In most difficult interactions, especially ones with our kids, we tend to fixate on the immediate and obvious behaviors: breaking rules, not listening, giving us attitude, or eye rolling. These exist at the very small tip of the iceberg. Understandably, this is where most of us get caught, and we end up pushing harder, debating, yelling, or having hurt feelings

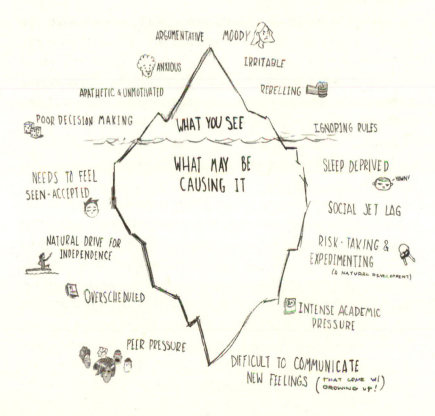

about all the overt behaviors that bother us. In so many instances, we are not really addressing what's truly going on in the much bigger part of the iceberg, below the surface.

That's because human psychology is too complex to express perfectly and directly all the time. Your teen's overt words and behaviors are only glimpses of the surface, which often cannot begin to show the vast and complex feelings and dynamics beneath the surface. When we get fixated on the tip of the iceberg, it often leads to an impasse in communication. The iceberg analogy helps us see past the obvious behaviors to what is really happening on a deeper level. When your teen does something that makes you bristle with frustration, remind yourself of the iceberg. Consider setting aside your immediate reaction and show curiosity about what they're really working on, struggling with, or experiencing. This does not mean you will let unacceptable behavior go or forget about family agreements (see Step 2: Limit-set), but it means you're the bigger person and you aren't going to take things personally or let your frustration get in the way of your caring. It's giving your teen the benefit of the doubt, communicating that you believe in her and will let her know this in an ongoing way. It can definitely feel like an act of faith, we know.

Having curiosity about what's under the tip of the iceberg naturally leads us to have more empathy for our kids rather than having feelings hurt on both sides, getting angry, or creating more distance. Even simply acknowledging there's more going on below the tip of the iceberg and *attempting* to understand allows our kids to lower their defenses and to feel less judgment from us (and toward themselves). This is the opening of the door leading to discussions, ideas, and collaboration that are at the very heart of turning conflict on its head. It opens space for your teens to uncover their own motivation, without which nothing will change. You are setting the stage for transforming impasses into growing, finding solutions, and supporting your teens in a way that is congruent with what is really going on beneath their surface behaviors.

SCENARIO ONE

Dad is struggling because his son is acting out, speaking in a rude way, and they're seemingly butting heads over everything. Dad keeps trying to address the rude tone and says, "Stop using that tone with me. I'm only trying to talk to you," or "Hey, that hurts my feelings." But the tone continues and it feels like they're growing apart.

Stepping back, Dad thinks about this behavior in another way. He realizes that what he and his son have lost, and may be mourning, is the joy of shared activities. Under the tip of the iceberg, his son is actually missing connection with his dad, something that has nothing to do with the daily responsibilities and comings and goings of everyday life. Like when his son was small and they used to sit and play Legos for an hour, uninterrupted. They've lost a common language. The son can't express it in a direct way (likely he doesn't even realize what's going on); his acting out is a sign of it, though.

Without saying why, Dad figures out what movie his son is dying to see and takes him. He suggests they walk to the theater instead of driving, and Dad purposefully calls out to everyone that he's leaving his phone, so if anyone needs him they'll have to wait. By the walk home, the two of them are laughing as they recount scenes from the movie, and they even chat about things they haven't in a long time. The negative tone dissolves, not because Dad addressed the tone directly, but because he addressed what was beneath the tip of the iceberg.

SCENARIO TWO

Imagine that Mom hears her eighteen-year-old son come home around 2:00 a.m. She's been lying awake, worried sick, and goes out to talk to him.

Mom: *Are you just coming in? You were supposed to be home hours ago!*

Son: *Never mind, you wouldn't understand. I didn't have a choice.*

Mom: *Of course you have a choice. You just decide to ignore the rules!*

Son: *I'm going to bed.* (Walks away.)

Again, the parent is stuck at the tip of the iceberg—what she sees on the surface. She feels worried and helpless, which makes her reactive. We all know how angry we can feel when we're fearful about our child's safety. We speak from that anger. There's no genuine or constructive communication, nor is there curiosity about what's really going on or what her son is feeling. She and her son are cut off from each other.

Now imagine this approach:

Mom: *Hi, are you just coming in? Is everything okay?*

Son: *Never mind, you wouldn't understand. I didn't have a choice.*

Mom: *Can you give me a try? I want to understand.*

Son: *Well, Mike and his girlfriend broke up and I didn't want to leave him alone. He's really messed up about it.*

Mom: *Wow, I'm really glad you told me. Poor guy. I get it and think you did the right thing to stay with him.*

Son: *Yeah, I didn't know what else to do.*

Mom: *The next time something like this happens, will you call or text me and let me know what's going on? It's really hard for me to lie awake worrying, not knowing if you're okay.*

Son: *I will. I guess I was afraid you'd just get mad and tell me to come straight home.*

Mom: *I will do my best to listen to what's going on with you and you can remind me if I don't. Should we have a code word for when I'm not getting it? Maybe "pineapple"?*

Son: *Haha. Okay. Pineapple. Night, Mom.*

Mom: *Do you need me to come up and tuck you in?*

Son: *Pineapple, Mom.*

In this example, the mom is curious about what's beneath the tip of the iceberg, what really happened, and asks her son to tell her more (and she even uses a little humor). Now she knows the details of the dilemma in which he found himself. Connecting with her son at this level of understanding creates an opening to make an agreement with him that he will communicate with her in the future, when things like this arise. Because she looked beneath the tip of the iceberg, he feels safe enough to do so. She also gave herself an opening to tell her son how she really feels (beneath the tip of *her* iceberg), scared rather than angry.

You won't always uncover what's really going on beneath the surface right away. That's okay. By listening to your teen and letting them know you want to understand, on a regular basis, you are building trust and kindness. Saying something like "I can tell something is up, and it's okay. I'm ready to listen anytime," you will make it easier for them to open up to you in the future.

PARENT ICEBERG

When we snap, yell, nag, or throw our hands up and walk away, we can usually feel that we're not having our best parenting moment. We feel disconnected, not only from our child but from what we are truly feeling. We can feel very alone in these moments. This happens because there's also more going on under the surface for us than we are aware of in the present moment. We all have our personal icebergs. In difficult moments with our kids, often what we're really feeling is fear. Fear that we're not doing a good job, fear that our child will not turn out okay, fear that being a parent is more than we know how to handle, or fear that we've failed or lost our connection to our kids. These are very normal and very painful fears. If we can connect the dots and look below the tip of our own parent iceberg, attuning to our worries and fears can help us to create more connection in the family. ALP works in all directions in relationships, including the one we have with ourselves.

Attune tool #3: The Good Waiter

We've all experienced bad service at a restaurant before. The waiter is distracted, disappears, or gets your order wrong. Sometimes, this is how we as parents must seem to our kids. On the other hand, a good waiter simply wants to get your order right, so he automatically listens carefully and paraphrases back (and we feel like, *Wow, he really gets me!*). Simply reflecting back what you hear or understand makes the other person feel acknowledged and not judged.

This is a key tool for increasing self-motivation, because it relates to your teen's experience, not your opinion, judgment, or expertise. It turns their attention to their own ideas instead of yours—and this is key to your teen developing his own motivation for healthy behaviors, including sleep. This technique works well when your teen is talking to you, expressing anything like a friend or school dilemma, how busy or overwhelmed or exhausted she is, or arguing all the reasons why she can't get more sleep. Stick to what she's telling you and resist adding your judgment, correction, or argument. Just paraphrase back what you heard.

Waiter:

So, you want the Caesar salad followed by the chicken special, and a sparkling water, is that right?

Mom to four-year-old:

I see. You're not feeling like washing your hands right now and you also want a snack?

Parents to teens:

You feel like you've got it under control.

Your practices and homework are really important to you.

You feel stuck and like there just isn't enough time for everything you want to do.

It feels like sleep is at the bottom of your list right now, is that right?

You really have a lot on your plate.

You're saying you are capable, but it seems to you like we don't trust you?

This feels like the most important thing at this moment.

If you start with your knee-jerk reaction, your teen is very likely to shut you out and feel alone with his dilemmas. By using the good waiter technique, you start from where your teen is and resist the temptation to judge, correct, or argue. It's a simple and powerful way to attune. He feels seen and heard, which is where empathy begins, and this opens the path to eventually finding solutions. This receptivity is key to staying connected and being seen as a helpful member of the team rather than as the contentious (and annoying!) opposition.

Here's an example of a conversation in which a dad resists the temptation to tell his daughter what to do, but instead continues to employ the good waiter:

Daughter: *I have so much to do, you don't understand!*

Dad: (Nods.) *I see that. You're really stretched.*

Daughter: *I'm doing everything I can, but there's no way I could get to bed earlier, it's just impossible.*

Dad: *It's like the day has no free space at all. You're jammed and you feel completely stuck.*

Daughter: *Yeah, practice is two hours, student council meetings, the times that I go on deliveries with the food bank, tutoring the fifth-grade kids, and then I took that job refereeing the basketball games... and that doesn't even include my homework!*

Dad: *It's so much just to juggle all those things—and then you still have hours of homework to do.*

Daughter: *I have too many things. They seem small at first, but then they add up.*

Dad: *Yeah, they seem good to take on in the moment, but when you put them all together...*

You can spot that the teen is starting to make the connections on her own. It might not happen right away, but she can tell she's overwhelmed, and she is starting to have some insight about how she got here and what her predicament is. In some cases, just your A step, employing the good waiter, is all you'll need, with the goal of helping your teen come to her own conclusions. In other cases, you'll want to follow it with an L and P step, which you'll see shortly.

The beauty of the good waiter technique is that by focusing on para-phrasing back what you heard your teen say, you are buying yourself time to notice and regulate your tendency to automatically react, judge, or give your own solutions. As psychotherapists, we were taught this skill in our first year of graduate school, but many people don't get the chance to practice this basic technique. The good waiter is an Empathy 101 strategy.

SELF-MOTIVATION: GETTING YOUR TEEN'S BUY-IN

If your teen isn't interested in sleeping better, simply giving advice is rarely an effective method. Adolescents often take this as being lectured to, and their resistance can increase or they just tune out. Researchers have seen that for teens, hearing advice from a parent often triggers unspoken counterarguments in their minds. This doesn't mean there's no place for you to offer your thoughts or to give your teen information. In fact, it's really important that you do—even if it *seems* like the information isn't landing, it is, trust us. It just means the ultimate goal is to help them identify their own motivation. Depending on the teen, this might be as simple as asking a few questions and relaying some data, while for others it might be a longer and more winding journey. Teenagers need autonomy, and they do not like to be bossed around or talked to as little kids. Many teens also like to learn about their own brains and bodies.

Look for an in as an opportunity to talk about sleep based on something they care about or complain about. For example:

"This math homework is so hard."
"My skin looks terrible."
"I keep getting injured."

You can also ask open-ended questions, imparting information in a way that is more helpful:

Instead of "Did you know that teens need nine to ten hours of sleep?"
Say, "Check out this one paragraph here."

Instead of "Do you think you get enough sleep?" or "Don't you think you need more sleep?"
Say, "How do you feel about your sleep?"

(continued)

225

Instead of "Do you think you need to go to bed earlier?"
Say, "What are your thoughts on when you go to bed and wake up?"

Instead of "You're tired, I can tell. Go to bed."
Say, "I saw you nodding off while we were watching a movie."

Instead of "Is your phone distracting you and keeping you up?"
Say, "What do you notice about your devices and your sleep?"

More open-ended questions and observations:

"I found this list of questions in this book, and I'm worried this is me. I'm sleep deprived!"
"Wow, reading this chapter about early high school start times—I didn't realize how hard this is on you guys. I feel kind of blown away, I wasn't aware."
"Who in this family wakes up feeling groggy?"
"Who in this family sometimes feels drowsy at the wheel?"
"How are you feeling today? I saw your light on really late last night."
"I know you think I'm overly concerned about sleep. Do you feel like it's not warranted?"
"What are some of the things that are important to you right now?"
"What are you enjoying most?"
"It's crazy, no one talked about this in school when I was a kid—people didn't realize that so much growing happens when you sleep. It basically shocked scientists when they figured out how much sleep helps kids your age."

Remember that for younger adolescents, it's still very reasonable and important to have set bedtimes and family agreements around phones, lights-out time, bedtime, and so forth. As we said in chapter 7, we often see parents let go of these rules too early because they see their teen asking for more independence. Independence is wonderful, but remember that the power and lure of technology is something no other teens of any generation had to contend with. Some teens need more support to balance this reality with their sleep.

Attune tool #4: The Sportscaster (not the referee)

The sportscaster is another tool for keeping communication open. It's a great way to stay neutral, convey attunement and understanding, gather facts—all the while resisting your knee-jerk reactions and giving you time to gather information. When something tricky happens or you're wondering what to say, describe what you see happening in front of you. You describe the play-by-play without making a judgment or jumping to conclusions. Just the facts, like a good sportscaster. While the good waiter paraphrases back what your teen is telling you, the sportscaster describes more generally what is happening in the moment, often between other people. Let's say you hear loud voices from the other room and you walk in to see your kids yelling at each other and a broken TV remote.

Knee-jerk response: *Hey, settle down! Which one of you did that?*

Sportscaster response: *Wow, something's up here. Really loud. You're both looking upset. I see a TV remote in pieces on the floor.*

You are gathering information and letting your kids know you see their struggles but you're not jumping to conclusions. As kids get older, we want to support them in solving their own conflicts, so sportscasting helps them feel as though you're there, but you're not necessarily going to give them the answer. If they need to be reminded of family agreements and rules, or need help solving problems, you will add your L and P steps.

Here's a mom using the sportscaster when she discovers her son, still awake, hours after bedtime.

> Mom: *Hi, honey. You're awake. I see your books and homework stuff out and your lights are on.*
>
> Son: *Yeah, I guess I lost track of the time.*
>
> Mom: *I know how that is. I also see your sleepy-looking eyes.*
>
> Son: *I actually drifted off a few times.*

This won't be the end of the conversation because Mom still has to hold the limit (L step) and support her son in coming up with a solution (P step). But what you can see here is how using the sportscaster opens the door to the son expressing that he lost track of the time and is very sleepy. This is huge. He's not defensive about how he's feeling, which helps him get in touch with his own motivation to make changes to his sleep habits. He feels like Mom is on his side rather than there to confront him.

Here's a dad, getting home from work to find his teenagers watching YouTube videos.

> Dad: *Hi, you two! What's up? I see my kids absorbed in some videos… unopened backpacks by the front door, and a dog who looks like she needs to go out.*
>
> Daughter: *Oops, we were just gonna watch one video my friend sent and then we got sucked in.*
>
> Son: *I was about to take April out and yeah, went right down the rabbit hole. Sorry, April, let me get your leash!*

In this example, Dad uses the sportscaster to help his kids become aware of their own behaviors and self-correct. They know what they are supposed to be doing and don't need to be nagged or chastised.

Attune tool #5: Join and use humor.

Have you ever sat down on the couch with a bowl of sour-cream-and-onion chips and watched *Minecraft* videos with your teenager, without rushing off to something else? If your teen will let you, you'll understand their point of view much better. Yes, you might not understand what's happening at all, but what better food for humor and self-deprecation? If you treat video games, social media, or online content as the enemy, it creates an adversarial dynamic. Instead, use tool number 5: Join in, use humor, and be on the same team.

Dig deep to find your humor and create a lighthearted tone in the house. Making a joke can instantly shift the tension in the air. It's not always called for, but imagine what would happen if, from time to time, instead of sighing or scolding, you tried (and yes, butchered) a TikTok dance near the TV to get your teen's attention. You have to know your teen and what makes them crack a smile, but don't be afraid to be silly, and don't be deterred by eye rolling. When we get into negative patterns, someone has to break the cycle, and you are the parent. Here are some more examples of good old-fashioned parent-humor:

Oh my goodness, my genius sweet daughter is being sucked away by YouTube! Where do I Like and Subscribe to folding up this laptop early, and watching a show together on the couch?

I know it's hard to shift gears and get ready for bed. When I was a kid, I used to read for hours by my night-light. Long ago, in a log cabin, listening to dinosaurs roam our front yard.

It's crazy, I'm as captured by my phone as you are. I find myself scrolling Instagram feeds that I'm not even interested in. Did you know there are accounts dedicated to hotel carpets?

Yikes, it's nine o'clock and there are absolutely no phones in the Good Night Box? Did the Good Night Box get robbed?! Should I call the phone police?

Hey, do they have a character in this game that runs out ten times to ask you to turn it off? Do they ever win? Just wondering what my odds are.

More homework, really? Which teacher gives the most homework? Whose house do we need to TP?

I know you think these blue-light-blocking glasses are dorky, but they seriously block a ton of laptop light. Now all I gotta worry about is the Cookie Monster sneaking up on me. Check me out!

Attune tool #6: Emotions as waves

Almost every single one of us can remember a moment when we felt completely overtaken by our emotions. A mom once described it as feeling like liquid anger was filling her entire body. A lovely and friendly teen once told us that when he felt angry he had the urge to throw things—in fact, in the moment he almost felt like he *had* to throw something to express the anger, as if it had to come out or he would burst. This peak in emotions subsides, though, and we almost always feel better with a little time.

Emotions as waves is a very helpful concept for teens and parents alike. Think of emotions as big waves and sometimes even storms. They wash over us, but the magnitude eventually fades. We always have our feelings throughout the day, but the difficult, intense ones are like summer rainstorms that open up from the skies and then pass.

Think of yourself as the boat captain who is navigating the complex waters of life, with your child as a VIP passenger (or co-captain, as they get older). You want to keep your eye on the horizon, take the long view, see the bigger picture, and not be thrown by the ups and downs of the water. You want to give your kids the sense that their feelings are normal, the intense emotions will subside, and we'll survive the difficult moments together. *This too shall pass.*

> *From Julie: When my son was a teen, I remember how many people told me, "He will circle back, trust me, it takes time." And they were right. For the teenage years, it can at times feel a bit like one long storm that parents will need to know is still going to pass. The bigger waves subside and come and go, while the one long storm will as well. It takes time and patience and holding on to ongoing unconditional love, not taking behaviors personally, being the bigger person, and keeping a sense of humor.*

When it comes to family routines and sleep habits, the Attune step is key to softening your teen's defenses so he can begin to connect the dots himself. Eventually, he'll link good sleep habits to his feelings of being more alert, positive, productive, and healthy. When he's not busy fighting or fleeing a parental response that is focused only on his surface behavior, and starts to feel truly understood without blame or shame, your teen will show you how much he really needs and welcomes an honest conversation about his struggles.

See page 242 for examples of all three ALP steps.

Step 2: Limit-set

ALP—Limit-setting: State the limit or rule, and briefly explain the reason.

Now that you've conveyed understanding in the Attune step, you're ready for Limit-setting. Limits will include your family agreements and rules of school and other outside entities, or any other boundaries you need to convey. This is why it's helpful to have regular family meetings in which you agree on limits, daily habits, responsibilities, and so forth. It makes the L step much easier, since you're starting from a common understanding.

When you state a limit, also give a brief reason for the limit. For example: "Screens need to go off because it's nine o'clock. Remember, YouTube wants you to stay up all night!" Giving the reason moves you from lawmaker to guide. You are helping your teen understand and gradually internalize the principles and morals behind your family's agreements and limits, leading to her inner sense of right and wrong. You are also treating her with a higher level of respect.

Setting reasonable limits continues to be something your teen needs from you when it comes to sleep habits, despite how vehemently hard he might push against them at times. Using your Parent Fade, you will adjust how you set limits as your adolescent matures. For young adolescents, you can clearly hold limits and rules around routines, screens, and bedtimes. In the later adolescent years, as your direct control over these aspects of life fades, you can shift toward appealing to your teen's self-motivation.

Before smart devices and the internet, it was much simpler for parents to hold on to sleep habits like regular bedtime, lights out, no TV in the bedroom, and so forth. Even if these rules were loose, we probably did okay as teens, because technology wasn't as powerful. When you were a teen, you may have stayed up late, talking on the phone with friends, listening to music, or watching TV. But that was nothing. The level of engagement and activation from devices and content today is exponentially higher; our experience with a landline in our bedroom or a boom box playing our favorite CDs does not compare.

We can't turn back time to those simpler days of long phone cords that wound around the house for us to talk on the phone, so as parents we have to work harder to hold the same limits. The incredibly alluring, even addictive nature of technology feels like an inevitable and unstoppable force sometimes. It's understandable to fear that your teen won't like you anymore if you have limits on when devices get docked for the night, lights out at an agreed-upon time, and so forth. But this won't happen. In fact, if you ask in a nonjudgmental way, most teens themselves will express needing limits around devices. We all do.

Limit-set tool #1: I know that you know

Let's face it, your teenager already knows most of the rules. Rather than simply stating a limit or family agreement that she already knows and is tired of hearing you repeat, try referring to it in a way that shows that you know that she knows: "Hey, I know you've got this already, but..." or "I know you know this..." You're less likely to sound like you're nagging or treating your teen like a little kid. Some teens will make this clear—"All you do is tell me what I already know! You talk to me like I'm a child or like I'm stupid"—while others will just roll their eyes and sigh. After many years of simply stating the rule or limit, this shift can be hard to remember at first. But it can really change the dynamic with your teen in a positive direction.

Limit-set tool #2: Turn a negative into a positive

It's more helpful to be told what we *can* do rather than what we *can't* do or what we're giving up. It's a good practice to remember this and give yourself a moment to turn your limit-setting statement into a positive rather than a negative. For example:

Negative limit: *Turn it off now, or I'm taking away a privilege.*

Positive limit: *Okay, looks like time is up, so let's take the dog on that run. Look at him staring at us—he knows it's time!*

Negative limit: *It's lights-out time, no more TV tonight.*

Positive limit: *It's lights-out time. Time to get cozy. We'll watch another episode tomorrow evening.*

Negative limit: *Hey, no more phone! It's past time for it to be in the charger.*

Positive limit: *Bud, look at the time. I do believe it's "shower and in bed with your book" time. I'm gonna do the same.*

It may feel like a subtle difference, but the psychological and emotional impact of stating a limit as a can-do and will-do is powerful.

Limit-set tool #3: Think beyond "Because I said so!"

Setting "Because I said so" limits won't get you to your long-term goals for your teen. We set limits as parents not to create mindlessly obedient kids but so that eventually they can make decisions from a higher level of principle (I do this because I know it's the right and good choice) rather than from blind adherence to authority (I do this because I've been told to do it and may be reprimanded or punished if I don't). Your goal is for your teenager to make good decisions when no one is around to monitor them and tell them what to do. This is what is meant by developing a moral compass.

Always explain the reason behind limits and rules. We're here to help teens develop a sense of right and wrong that they carry with them into the world. Our goal is to develop critical thinkers.

Adding an explanation in your limit is also a respectful way to communicate to anyone. You probably wouldn't tell a friend or peer what to do without explaining why. For example:

We don't bring our phones to the table at mealtimes because it's one of the few times we come together as a family and it's our time to check in with one another.

We do the "work before play" thing because it's so much more satisfying to play once our work is done.

We put phones and other tech into their chargers outside the bedroom an hour-p2.14 before bed because this gets our body and brain prepared to fall asleep easily at bedtime.

Doing homework while also watching YouTube is like running two channels at once. Promise, it really crosses brain signals.

Limit-set tool #4: Limit your nos

Do you find yourself saying no a lot? If so, consider swapping it with other phrases. Here's why:

- The word "no" triggers automatic resistance.
- Saying no is a conversation ender. It can crush communication.
- Saying no over and over will usually end up being ignored, like you're talking to the wall.
- Saying no doesn't contain details or an explanation.
- Saying no is negative (clearly). Using the can-do version of the limit sets a more positive tone.
- No doesn't acknowledge what your teen already knows and is likely to evoke feelings of "You treat me like a five-year-old!"
- No, on its own, can feel shaming and needlessly harsh.

You can still communicate a limit that is clear and firm. Limiting nos just means that you'll work on using language that connects you and your teen and helps to keep communication open.

Limit-set tool #5: State the reality

In many moments, there isn't a limit or rule to state, but rather a "reality." In these cases, the reality step can help you impart a little wisdom or just help your teenager accept, well, reality.

Here's the earlier conversation between the dad and his high-achieving teenage daughter. But now Dad states the reality as well, which ends up being helpful:

Daughter: *I have so much to do, you don't understand!*

Dad: (Nods.) *I see that. You're really stretched.*

Daughter: *I'm doing everything I can, but there's no way I could get to bed earlier. It's just impossible.*

Dad: *It's like the day has no free space at all. You're jammed and you feel completely stuck.*

Daughter: *Yeah, practice is two hours, student council meetings, the times that I go on deliveries with the food bank, tutoring the fifth-grade kids, and then I took that job refereeing the basketball games . . . and that doesn't even include my homework!*

Dad: *It's so much just to juggle all those things—and then you still have hours of homework to do.*

Daughter: *I have too many things. They seem small at first, but then they add up.*

Dad: *Yeah, they seem good to take on in the moment, but when you put them all together . . .*

Daughter: *Yeah.*

Dad: *I know you already know this, but sometimes it's easy to forget. It's better to do a few things well and really enjoy them. You don't have to do everything at once.*

Daughter: *Yeah.*

Dad: (With a smile.) *It's a thought.*

See page 242 for examples of all three ALP steps.

Scenario: Your teen came in past curfew.	
Attune	I heard you come in at twelve thirty last night. What was going on?
Limit-set	You already know this, but curfew isn't negotiable until school's out for the summer. Then we can talk again. Curfew is a way to make sure you're safe and to protect your sleep.
Scenario: Your teen is still on her phone after you've asked repeatedly for her to put it away.	
Attune	Hey, I know it feels impossible to put it down. Believe me, I feel it myself sometimes.
Limit-set	It's time to help with dinner prep. You know where phones go until after we're done eating.
Scenario: Your twelve-year-old is still playing a video game after you've said turn it off.	
Attune	You feel like you can't stop, huh? What level are you on? Ah, cool.
Limit-set	It's time to turn it off because we're going to your sister's game.
Scenario: Your teen is up late, past bedtime.	
Attune	I know you're saying you don't need more sleep. I also see you struggling a bit and not feeling your best sometimes.
Limit-set	The family bedtimes we agreed on are still in place because, as you know, sleeping well helps with just about everything.
Scenario: You have to wake your teen ten times before she gets out of bed.	
Attune	It's really hard for you to wake up in the morning. It's like you feel like you're so deeply asleep and dreaming. I know the feeling.
Reality step	It's not a good use of my time because I'm getting ready for work. I need to hand this job over to you. I'm on the committee to move school start times later, but for now, it is what it is. I don't like it any more than you do, but while we wait on the school to act, we have to make the best of it.

Scenario: Your teen has his phone in his room past the agreed-on time.	
Attune	I get it, it's hard to find time to hang with your friends when you get home from practice at six and have so much homework to do.
Limit-set	It's nine o'clock. Remember we agreed on a time for parking phones so we make space for sleeping.
Scenario: Your young teen is still on his computer late at night.	
Attune	You've got so much you have to do—and so much you *want* to do—I really see that. It's hard to shut it down.
Limit-set	It's getting late, and you've gotta give your eyes and your brain a break so you can sleep. Pop your computer into the office, where it goes at night.
Scenario: You're trying to ask your teen a question and he yells at you unexpectedly.	
Attune	*Pause.* Wow, okay, something's bothering you.
Limit-set	It really feels pretty terrible being talked to that way. I'm not okay with it.

Step 3: Problem-solve

ALP—Problem-solve: Support your teen in coming up with acceptable or more helpful alternatives or solutions.

WHICH IS BETTER, REWARDS OR PUNISHMENTS? NEITHER.

When it comes to enforcing rules, emotions and disbelief can sometimes run high when we suggest letting go of rewards and punishments. But let's look at why we'd suggest getting rid of such classic parenting tools. What is a punishment? The definition of a punishment is making a person suffer for something they did. Sometimes people think punishments are simply "just," as in the person deserves to suffer for a bad action. Sometimes people think punishments serve the purpose of teaching the person not to do it again (this is more likely the case for parents). But both of these lines of reasoning have a very negative view of kids, and we definitely do not want our teens to get these messages about themselves. Punishments tell our kids we do not believe they have good intentions. We've "caught" them, we don't think they want to do the right or good thing, and we aren't curious about what happened or how they may need different support from us. Punishments make people feel ashamed and act out of fear of getting caught. Punishments have been shown by multiple research studies to stop people from being able to think creatively and to shut down problem-solving and new ideas.

If you're wondering how you would possibly hold sway or power in your home without punishments, we'd like to challenge you to reframe your thinking. Instead of trying to exert power or control, think about trying to understand what's really going on, and consider yourself a guide. You can be a clear and steady navigator, without using threats and punishments. You are on the same side, believing in the desire and tendency of your child or teen to be a good human, figure out the world within safe limits, make mistakes, and grow her moral compass (not just the view you have given to her, but the views she genuinely grows from the inside out).

Let's consider an example: Your son is mean to his younger brother. At a certain point, you might feel frustrated and say, "I told you to be nice to each other. You can't be mean like that. If you don't stop it, I'm taking away your phone. And you're not play-ing video games this weekend." First of all, the punishment that is being threatened has nothing to do with the action of being mean to the brother—it's an unrelated consequence, so it doesn't really make sense. But more important, it doesn't help you uncover any-thing about why the brother is being mean, what he's really trying to express, how to help the younger brother set his own limits and stand up for himself—it shuts down communication and doesn't

(continued)

239

facilitate the brothers' understanding each other so they can get along better. This kind of "tip of the iceberg" threatening can keep siblings feeling distant and resentful of each other.

Rewards can also miss the mark. As researcher and author Alfie Kohn writes, rewards and punishments are not opposites, they're two sides of the same coin, and both are based on manipulation. Rewards have been shown in many studies to decrease our intrinsic motivation to do something (we do it for the carrot being dangled in front of us, not the interest or joy), to make kids give up, and to reduce creativity and risk-taking. As an example we see repeatedly in our sleep consulting practice, parents often tell us they've "tried everything" to get their preschooler to stay in bed all night, including sticker charts that lead to a big prize at the end of the week for compliance. Not surprisingly, most three-year-olds will do this for a night or two—or maybe stick it out for a week to cash in on the trip to the toy store—but the effect fades and they're back to jumping out of bed. On top of that, the inherent message is that sleep is the bad guy, the dreaded spear of broccoli that must be eaten before dessert (when we all know broccoli is yummy and sleep is luxurious). We inadvertently send kids the wrong message about all kinds of wonderful and enjoyable activities when we reward the joy out of them.

What to do instead? Use the steps of ALP to address difficult moments. Natural consequences can be helpful. For example, if your teen is unable to turn off her phone at the agreed-on time despite multiple attempts to address the issue, you might have to step in and take the phone before bedtime for a while (or find a creative solution like parental controls or shutting down the internet, which we've heard parents tell us they do). This is not to make her suffer—this is because she's showing you she isn't able to stay within the agreements and needs support for sticking to the limit and behaving in a safe and healthy way.

To be clear, not using punishments and rewards does not mean you are a permissive parent. You are there to teach, guide, and hold reasonable limits—but always approaching your child from the point of view that they are good, empathic, creative, and capable human beings trying to navigate the world. When they do something that you don't like, or break a rule, they are telling you they need your help with something and need you to be on their team. Seeing your child this way means they will see themselves this way too.

You've conveyed understanding with the Attune step and communicated a rule or reality with the Limit-setting step. Now support your teen in coming up with a path forward—a way to solve the dilemma in an acceptable way. The Problem-solving step is where you work together with your teen to find an alternative solution. The P step is hopeful, creative, and collaborative. It can also be fun and lighthearted at times. It's a chance to think outside the box and explore ways for your teen to fulfill their intentions while still following the rule or family agreement.

The trickiest part of this step is how tempting it is to just tell your teen what to do, remembering how much better that probably worked when they were younger. The key to problem-solving with teens is that ultimately they need to feel like part (and eventually all) of the solution-creating process and that they have a choice among options. This doesn't mean we don't hold reasonable limits consistently, but rather that if your teen isn't invested in the outcome, your well-intended ideas will meet with resistance and a shutdown of communication.

Teens' drive to become progressively more independent is illustrated in a very exciting way in this step. The path to solving problems while keeping family bonds tight and loosening the reins gradually is finding out what they really want, what motivates them, and listening to their ideas with an open mind and heart. Your teen is full of creative energy—this is the time to celebrate it.

Scenario: Your teen came in past curfew.	
Attune	I heard you come in at twelve thirty last night. What was going on?
Limit-set	You already know this, but curfew isn't negotiable until school's out for the summer. Then we can talk again. Curfew is a way to make sure you're safe and to protect your sleep.
Problem-solve	Did you like the idea of me or Mom texting you a code word so you can tell your friends you got a text and gotta go? You don't have to tell them the text was from your boring old parents (unless it's easier to blame it on us!). My parents actually did something like this with me, back in the day, on a landline if you can believe it. Once you're following your curfew consistently, we wouldn't have to do this anymore. Or maybe you have another idea.
Scenario: Your teen is still on her phone after you've asked repeatedly for her to put it away.	
Attune	Hey, I know it feels impossible to put it down. Believe me, I feel it myself sometimes.
Limit-set	It's time to help with dinner prep. You know where phones go until after we're done eating.
Problem-solve	Your choice: Should we listen to music, the news, or a podcast while we make dinner?
Scenario: Your twelve-year-old is still playing a video game after you've asked him to turn it off.	
Attune	You feel like you can't stop, huh? What level are you on? Ah, cool.
Limit-set	It's time to turn it off because we're going to your sister's game.
Problem-solve	I know you don't like when I yell to turn it off because your friends can hear me. I'm going to write you a note and hold it up. If that doesn't work, though, I have to just turn it off myself, which I don't like doing!

Scenario: Your teen is up late, past bedtime.	
Attune	I know you're saying you don't need more sleep. I also see you struggling a bit and not feeling your best sometimes.
Limit-set	The family bedtimes we agreed on are still in place because, as you know, sleeping well helps with just about everything.
Problem-solve (younger adolescent)	Do your last thing, and I'll come back and check on you in ten minutes so we can turn the lights out and chat a little.
Problem-solve (older adolescent)	I could see that you were awake much later than your bedtime last night. I'm wondering if there's something you could take off your crazy-busy schedule? What do you think? Let me know how I can help.
Scenario: You have to wake your teen ten times before she gets out of bed.	
Attune	It's really hard for you to wake up in the morning. It's like you feel like you're so deeply asleep and dreaming. I know the feeling.
Reality step	It's not a good use of my time because I'm getting ready for work. I need to hand this over to you. I'm on the committee to move school start times later, but for now, it is what it is. I don't like it any more than you do, but while we wait on the school to act, we have to make the best of it.
Problem-solve	Pick out any non-light-up alarm clock you want with a reasonable price, and I'll get it for you. I'm getting one for your sister too. This way, none of us will need our phones to use as an alarm. There's a cool one I saw that simulates the sun rising.
Scenario: Your teen has his phone in his room past the agreed-on time.	
Attune	I get it, it's hard to find time to hang with your friends when you get home from practice at six and have so much homework to do.
Limit-set	It's nine o'clock. Remember, we agreed on a time for parking phones so we make space for sleeping.
Problem-solve	The last time we talked about this, you mentioned setting an alert fifteen minutes before nine o'clock to help you remember. Do you still like that idea? How about if, as a family, we all set that alert so we're parking phones at the same time, and then meet for a quick snack or good-night chat? It's like we need a bugle to play taps like they used to do at camp, so we feel like we're all in it together! Any other ideas?

Scenario: Your young teen is still on his computer late at night.	
Attune	You've got so much you have to do—and so much you *want* to do—I really see that. It's hard to shut it down.
Limit-set	It's getting late, and you've gotta give your eyes and your brain a break so you can sleep. Pop your computer into the office, where it goes at night.
Problem-solve	Let's talk about it tomorrow, but it seems like doing homework first thing when you get home might help, so it's not getting pushed into the evening when you like to do fun stuff. Let's figure out what schedule works for you.
Scenario: You're trying to ask your teen a question and he yells at you unexpectedly.	
Attune	*Pause.* Wow, okay, something's bothering you.
Limit-set	It really feels pretty terrible being talked to that way. I'm not okay with it.
Problem-solve	Let me know when you want to talk. I'd love to hear what's underneath all this.

Here's the dad and his daughter continuing to talk about schedules. Now that Dad has done his A and L steps, see where he adds a Problem-solving step:

Daughter: *I have so much to do, you don't understand!*

Dad (Attune): (Nods.) *You're really stretched.*

Daughter: *I'm doing everything I can, but there's no way I could get to bed earlier. It's all impossible.*

Dad: *It's like the day has no free space at all. You're jammed and you feel completely stuck.*

Daughter: *Yeah, practice is two hours, student council meetings, the times that I go on deliveries with the food bank, tutoring the fifth-grade kids, and then I took that job refereeing the basketball games . . .*

Dad: *It's so much.*

Daughter: *I have too many things. They seem small at first, but then they add up.*

Dad: *They seem good to take on in the moment, but when you put them all together...*

Daughter: *Yeah.*

Dad (Limit-set): *I know you already know this, but sometimes it's easy to forget. It's better to do a few things well and really enjoy them. You don't have to do everything at once.*

Daughter: *Yeah.*

Dad (Problem-solve): *It's a thought. Of all the stuff you're doing, what do you enjoy most?*

Daughter: *I kinda love refereeing those games, funny enough. I look forward to it more than the tutoring.*

Dad: *You could focus on that for a bit and put tutoring on hold, I guess?*

Daughter: *That sounds better, actually.*

Problem-solve tool #1: The Bumbling Parent

This is the moment when you put a lid on all the great ideas you're dying to lay out to your teen in the futile hope that miraculously, she will say, "Hey, Mom, that's a great idea, I'll do that!" It's far more likely that you trying to take over and fix things is not at all what your teen wants or needs. Instead, furrow your brow, metaphorically scratch your head, and say something like "Hmmm, thinking... Don't have a solution right now" or "Not sure what would help with this" or "Nothing's coming to me right now. What do you think?"

Keep the ball in your teen's court as much as possible. He is much more likely to come up with a creative solution if 1) he's not being told what to do, 2) he has the sense that you believe in his ability to find a solution, and 3) he feels the satisfaction of being better than you at knowing what will work best for him. With the bumbling parent, you are not throwing limits and rules out the window (you maintain your Limit-setting step), but now you're figuring out how to move forward.

The beauty of the bumbling parent is that you are making space for your teen's natural desire to be her own person and make her own decisions.

BUMBLING PARENT CONVERSATION

Honey, just a heads-up that it's almost eleven o'clock (this family's agreed-upon bedtime for both parents and teens).

Dad, I just finished my homework, but I still have to shower and empty the dishwasher.

(Attune step) *Must feel good to have your homework done. Haven't gotten to shower and do your chores, huh?*

(Limit-setting step) *Well, you know the deal.*

(Problem-solving step—bumbling parent) *Hmmm, not sure what the answer is. You'll come up with something.*

The next morning:

Good morning! Hey, I noticed the dishwasher is empty and (sniff, sniff) *you smell pretty clean. How'd you do that?*

Took one of my three-minute showers last night and set my alarm three minutes earlier this morning to do the dishwasher.

Ah, nice idea. Wish I could be as speedy as you!

Problem-solve tool #2: You've got this

Teenagers are just as good as adults at coming up with ideas and solutions to problems, and the truth is that as much as we'd like to swoop in with the answer, it's not helpful for us to do so. Similar to the bumbling parent, this means that the Problem-solving step will often be expressed as our confidence in our teens' ability to solve the problem. For example:

I bet you'll get to the bottom of this.

I know you'll figure it out.

Do you have a plan?

It's a tough one. Let me know if you wanna brainstorm ideas.

Problem-solve tool #3: Use humor

If you choose your moments, humor can provide an excellent way to change the channel from adversarial or stuck to a more lighthearted, "We can get through this" kind of spirit. Both parents and teens can feel a sense of relief when you surprise them with something absurd or silly.

Finding ways to inject humor in the Problem-solving step will take some creativity. It's not appropriate for every difficult moment. It's also really important to be careful not to ever mock or make fun of your child. Here are a few ideas. Heather's daughter points out that from time to time, even a "Dad joke" works.

Okay, I'm putting everyone's phones, including mine, into the microwave for the night with a bright piece of tape securing them. No breaching the tape until six a.m.!

I'm going to stand on my head until we come up with a solution here!

Oh my, this laundry is so nice and warm. I'll just put it here (on top of your teen) *so I can fold it.*

How about we move to a desert island where we don't have to worry about jobs and homework and texts and emails and blah, blah, blah!

Often, you'll find that the humor step opens the door for true problem-solving to emerge. We all let down our guard and gain perspective with a little well-placed humor and then are able to think creatively about what we *can* do to solve a dilemma.

Problem-solve tool #4: Parent "calm-down" time

In our book *Now Say This*, which is a guide to using ALP with babies and kids, we teach "calm-down" time rather than "time-out" as a way of truly helping children, instead of isolating and punishing them, when they are having a hard time. We also recommend parents use "calm-down" time for themselves—a strategy that can work well with older kids and teens, especially during an escalating, heated, or argumentative conversation. Say, "I'm feeling a little overwhelmed [triggered, emotional, stuck, or whatever fits]. I'm going to take a little calm-down time. I'll be back in twenty minutes." Slowly walk into another room, ideally one where you can close the door (quietly). Use the time to breathe deeply and center yourself in any way you like. Be kind and empathic with yourself—turn the Attune step inward to understand and accept yourself.

After twenty minutes, go back to your teen and check in. Repeat the Attune step for each of you, holding off repeating the limit and reasons why (your teen already knows) and see if you can get beyond the stuck place. What you'll often find is that the eye of the storm passes during your twenty-minute calm-down time: high-intensity emotions can lower in as little as ninety seconds. Now you and your teen are better able to listen to each other with kindness and collaborate on a solution. What parents tend to find with this tool is that their child will come to them before the twenty minutes are over, ready to talk. It shifts the dynamic in a way that helps your teen see and hear and listen to you (have empathy for you) as well. It's very important that the parent calm-down is not carried out in an angry, huffy, "I can't stand to be near you" way. You're not judging or punishing; you're just taking a break. You're modeling that effective communication can happen only when we are present and calm.

Repair and Circle Back

As you're beginning to put these steps into practice, go easy on yourself. Think of it as a quest, a journey, a climb toward the peak of a very tall mountain. We never get to the very top, but the act of climbing toward it, of trying to remember to lead with empathy (the Attune step is the most commonly forgotten), is more than enough.

None of us gets this right all the time. If you did, that would be weird and you'd be a robotically perfect parent—which is not helpful to your child. When you forget to lead with empathy, when you lose your cool and yell or argue or when you throw up your hands and give up, you have actually created an opportunity. It's called "repair" and it means that you now have a chance to circle back to that difficult moment, later that day or the next day, and talk about it with your teen. You have a chance to apologize for yelling or giving up and to say the attuned, empathic thing you wish you had said the first time. You can ask for a "do-over" or you can say how you'd like to handle it differently the next time. In preparation for future difficult moments, you can give your teen permission to say, "Hey, Mom, remember you said you'd start by trying to understand things from my point of view?" You can also calmly ask for the same understanding from him, describing how you were feeling in the heat of the moment.

An amazing mom shared with us that, in the middle of an argument with her young adolescent, she'd stop and say, "You know what? I don't like how we're talking to each other. I don't like how my voice is getting louder. I love and respect you. Can we start over and try again?" The daughter would always say yes, calm down, and they'd start over. After a couple of times doing this, she came to her mom once during a meltdown, hugged her, and said, "Mom, can we start over?" Of course her mom hugged her and said yes. It felt like a revelation.

By presenting ourselves to our kids as imperfect human beings, which of course we all clearly are, we are helping them accept themselves as imperfect. Being fallible is perfectly normal and how we learn. We are showing them that life will always have its bumps and bruises and that it helps a lot to be able to talk about them. Listening carefully to each other almost always takes the drama and heat out of the situation, leaving us feeling relieved and in a much better place to find solutions. By turning what you may think of as a failure into a chance to connect more genuinely and honestly with your teen, you are modeling for him how to navigate difficult relational moments throughout his life. You're willing to admit when you've made a mistake, and now he feels safer doing the same when he's made a mistake. You build his trust in you and his feeling that he is safe with you, even in vulnerable situations.

9

The Sleep Challenge

Before we part ways and you head off to bed, remember this: sleeping well at night is the elixir you need to transform your day.

And while we're serious about sleep—this subject we love so much—we're also human. We realize that sleep advice can sound like homework—a list of to-dos that often involve taking away enjoyable habits (electronics, caffeine, staying up late . . .) that we feel attached to. Every so often, a slightly glazed look appears on a client's face as we make suggestions (especially if it involves disrupting something like a coveted TV-in-bed habit). It's a weary look that says, "Oh, please don't take *that* away from me. I can't!"

But the truth is, you can. Just ten or twenty years ago—a mere blip on the human time scale—none of us were streaming YouTube from our bedrooms or scrolling through social media in the middle of the night. So the idea that we can't do it is a myth (one that tech companies are quite happy to support). Sleep emerged millions of years ago, and it doesn't understand or care about the tantalizing offerings of our modern world. Nature will not, and should not, adapt to Netflix—it must be the other way around. To improve sleep, we have to better sync our habits to the natural world.

Taking steps to protect your sleep—especially managing technology, creating sleep-conducive "cave" environments, having routines and regular timing, and advocating for healthy high school schedules—is within your reach. And every step you take leads to fifteen or thirty minutes more sleep, which leads to replenishing precious minutes of sleep's vital work. Those thirty minutes, over time, could change the course of a teenager's life.

It's easy to dismiss sleep because we don't consciously experience it. If we did, we'd see a spectacular symphony of memory formation, emotional balancing, muscle strengthening, hormone secretion, and more happening in front of our eyes. If we could watch what sleep does, there's no way any of us would skimp on it. We would fully appreciate good sleep as the overnight magic that it is. This should remind all of us of our bigger purpose in advocating, as a society, to protect our teenagers' sleep—and with it, their mental and physical health. When we do this, we're boosting the happiness, safety, and well-being of families and our communities as a whole.

THE SLEEP CHALLENGE:
YOUR ORGANIZING TOOL

We sure do know a whole lot about sleep, but what we don't know are all the details of your life in particular. What's your high school start time? How long is your commute and do you ride the bus, walk, ride your bike, or ride in a car? How much time does it take to get home from school, do your homework, and complete any jobs or after-school activities you have? What is important to you—good grades, being in shape, helping your family, feeling positive and energetic? This Sleep Challenge tool is a way for you to personalize what you've learned, write down your own information, and create routines, timing, and goals to motivate you. We know from experience working with clients that having a comprehensive plan and visualizing our motivations for change is key.

It's important to read chapter 6 so that you understand the underlying mechanisms of the five sleep habits and the concepts of paleo-sleep and the sleep bubble. The Sleep Challenge in this chapter is solely focused on helping you put all you've learned together into your own unique plan. You may choose to take the steps of the Sleep Challenge on your own, with a friend, with your family, your class, or an athletic team. It's a great idea to do it together so you can brainstorm and troubleshoot, check in and hold one another accountable. Whether it's with family, friends, or on your own, remember you are committing to prioritizing your sleep, rather than letting it get shuffled to the bottom of the list. You're moving from a sleep-comes-last to a sleep-forward mentality.

On our website, thehappysleeper.com, you will find more tools, along with a printable version of the sleep challenge.

STEP ONE: THE SETUP

The first step is to answer the following questions so you get a baseline on your quantity and quality of sleep. You'll identify what's getting in your way, and you'll lay out the reasons why (read: motivation!) you want to get better sleep. This is to assess where you are. Don't overthink these questions. Answer them without worrying or judging yourself.

MEASURE YOUR SLEEP AND SLEEPINESS

Write down the amount of sleep you get during an average week, based on the time you fall asleep and what time you wake up. The time you fall asleep is likely an estimate, since most of us don't know exactly. If it changes between weekend and weekday, note that too.

Most weeknights I sleep from _____ to _____, total sleep time: _____
Saturday nights I sleep from _____ to _____, total sleep time: _____
Sunday nights I sleep from _____ to _____, total sleep time: _____

As a reminder, here's how much sleep, in hours, we need:

Little kids (2–6): 12–13
Big kids (7–11): 10–12
Adolescents (12–18): 9–10 (Remember, 8–8.5 may be *adequate* and
     9–10 is *optimal*)
Adults: 7–9

Next, if your sleep times are lower than the recommended range, or if there is more than one hour of difference between your weeknight and weekend sleep time, note this.

I need _____ more sleep each night
I sleep _____ more on the weekends or vacations

(Sleeping one to two hours more on the weekend versus the weeknights indicates sleep debt during the week and contributes to social jet lag.)

Which of these statements do you agree with?

____ I find it hard to wake up and get out of bed on school days.
____ If I lie down, sit down in class, or am riding to school as a passenger in the car or on the bus, I could fall asleep.
____ I find it hard to focus in class and my mind wanders.

___ If I put my head on my desk at school, I could fall asleep.

___ It takes me longer to do my homework than I'd like.

___ I feel bored at school or like I'm in a daze.

___ I fall asleep when I get home from school.

___ If I get to bed on time, it's hard for me to fall asleep.

While not a clinical assessment tool, if you answer yes to some of these questions, it's likely that you need more sleep. Put together, the amount of sleep you get each night, along with these signs of inadequate sleep, will help you see if you need to add more sleep to your nightly schedule.

Ideally, I should get _____ hours of sleep each night.

During the week, my schedule should be:

Bedtime _____

Wake time _____

On the weekend or school holidays, my schedule should be:

Bedtime _____

Wake time _____

(Aim to keep your weekend schedule within one or two hours of your weekday schedule.) For more on this dilemma of sleeping in, see page 153.

UNDERSTAND THE PERFECT STORM SO YOU CAN STAY OUT OF ITS PATH

What is making it hard for you to get optimal sleep? Our modern world makes sleep very difficult. Sleep is often a last priority when all the things in the day are done. Check the factors that are impacting your sleep:

Smartphones and the difficulty of saying goodbye/good night to
friends

Difficulty turning off video games or online content

Overscheduling

Noise or light pollution

Academic overload

Job responsibilities

Stress or anxiety

Worry about safety or the future

Difficulty winding down and falling asleep (often due to home lighting, screens, and social jet lag)

Too-early school start times

Long commute/transportation issues

Undervaluing sleep

What else can you add? _____

Since technology is one of our main "sleep stealers," look at page 101
in chapter 4. Ask these questions out loud to your family or friends and
let them be your guide for talking about how technology affects us and
the power it has over our sleep.

CHALLENGE MYTHS

Circle any of the following myths that you see around you or that apply
to your own thinking. Select those you think might be affecting you, and
rewrite them to reflect a more helpful and sleep-forward view. (This is an
exercise in cognitive behavioral therapy—often cited as having the highest evidence-based efficacy.) For example, "If I stay up late and cram, I'll
do better on my tests" might become "Studying incrementally and getting enough sleep means my brain remembers information and I'll do
even better on my tests."

My sleep can wait. I can tough it out.

_____

I don't need as much sleep as other people. (This is a common myth, when in fact a very small percentage of the population needs less sleep than the rest of us.)

_____

If I stay up late and cram, I'll do better on my tests.

_____

I must get into the best-ranked college to be happy.

_____

I have to do lots of AP classes and after-school activities for my college applications.

_____

I should try to be good at everything.

_____

I need to know what's going on in the world at all times.

_____

I need to know what my friends are doing at all times.

_____

I have to respond to texts and alerts immediately.

_____

Bedtime routines are just for babies and little kids.

_____

IDENTIFY YOUR *WHY*

By now you know the myriad benefits of good sleep, but it helps to identify the benefits you personally would like to achieve. Really go long on this list and search out your own personal truths of why you want to live a better life. It doesn't matter if they relate to health or even what people would consider superficial things. (Heather's husband cites how much better he looks on Zoom when he's sleeping well.) These reasons should be what matters to you—no matter what they are—and they will be your motivation. When you have the thought "Lemme just skim Instagram in bed real quick," this list is your motivational coach yelling, "Leave that goshdarn phone behind so we can shave time off that 400 meter dash!" Do not start your challenge without this step! For the challenge to work, you should think about what it is you wish for, not what your partner or parent says is important. If you don't feel connected to *why* you are doing something, it's harder to stick with it.

Choose the benefits you would like to acquire in your life, along with the corresponding negative effects of inadequate sleep you would like to say goodbye to. Choose at least two from the following chart.

ADEQUATE SLEEP LEADS TO:		TOO LITTLE SLEEP LEADS TO:
Positive mood/outlook	vs.	Feeling down/pessimistic
Ability to focus	vs.	Poor focus/concentration
Good energy level	vs.	Low energy/lethargic
Improved appearance	vs.	Looking tired, dark circles
Physical strength/athleticism	vs.	Lower strength/athletic ability
More patient/longer fuse	vs.	Short-tempered
Weight normalizes	vs.	Weight gain
Improved immune function	vs.	Low immune strength
Overall health benefits	vs.	Long-term health problems

ADEQUATE SLEEP LEADS TO:		TOO LITTLE SLEEP LEADS TO:
Better relationships	vs.	Relationship conflicts
Depression/anxiety lessen	vs.	Depression/anxiety increase
_____	vs.	_____
_____	vs.	_____

STEP TWO: CLARIFY YOUR GOAL

What exactly do you want to change or improve in regard to your sleep? You've gathered good info from Step 1. Now put it together here. This could be as simple as increasing your sleep time by half an hour, improving your routines, or creating more technology boundaries—they are all interwoven. Your goal is not necessarily the same as anyone else's—friends, parents, siblings, and so forth. Articulate your goal in your own words. We're both fans of achievable goals. This isn't about being perfect—this is about doing what works in your life.

For example:

I want to sleep thirty minutes more every school night.

I will put my phone away each night in another room so I can feel more peaceful.

I am going to wake up on the weekends by 8:30 a.m. to reduce my social jet lag.

My goal is to fall asleep easier.

My goal is to reduce my stress levels and sleep one hour more each school night.

STEP THREE: MODIFY YOUR 5 SLEEP HABITS

No matter your unique goal, the five habits will help you achieve it. The good news is that the habits work together and all contribute to creating a sleep bubble. But this also means that, since they work together, we cannot leave one out—the bubble could lose air or even pop. For example, if you set good bedtimes, but you don't put away electronics an hour before, you sleep in too late on Sunday, or you nap in the late afternoon after school one day—the good bedtime habit is likely to suffer. All of the five habits support one another, so addressing each of them is super important. Sorry, we'd love to have you pick and choose, but nature did not form our finely tuned biological sleep systems this way! It doesn't mean that you have to be strict about every single piece of gold standard information, but if you're not sleeping enough and feeling your best, this is your body telling you to take a step closer to that gold standard.

The Five Habits of Happy Sleepers:

1. S—Set your sleep times
2. L—Lay out your three routines
3. E—Extract your sleep stealers; replace unhelpful sleep associations with helpful ones
4. E—Eliminate light and make your bedroom a cave
5. P—Practice a sleep-friendly daytime

HABIT #1: SET YOUR SLEEP TIMES

Using the information on page 154, write down your new sleep and wake times. To give your regular bedtime the prelude it needs, remember your wind-down begins sixty minutes before sleep. Wind-down is simple; the only *must-dos* are putting away certain devices, turning off bright lights in the house, and creating a calm feeling. Your bedtime routine can start about fifteen to thirty minutes before your bedtime.

My sleep times

WEEKDAY	WEEKEND
Wind-down _____	Wind-down _____
Bedtime routine _____	Bedtime routine _____
Sleep _____	Sleep _____
Wake time _____	Wake time _____

Instead of jumping to a new bedtime, move your sleep times fifteen to thirty minutes longer per night until you get to the right time. If possible, keep your weekend bedtime and wake time within an hour of your weekday times. In the examples below, see that the younger teen is able to move toward optimal sleep, while the older teen's realistic goal is adequate sleep during the school week.

Examples:

- A twelve-year-old who goes to sleep at 10:30 p.m. and wakes at 6:30 a.m. is getting eight hours and is missing one to two hours per night (for optimal sleep). Her goal is to increase her nightly sleep by one hour. The first week, she moves her bedtime thirty minutes earlier, to 10:00 p.m.—putting away all devices at 9:00 p.m.—and she sets her alarm fifteen minutes later in the morning, as she doesn't have to leave the house until 7:30 a.m. The second week she moves her bedtime to 9:45 p.m. Now she's sleeping from 9:45 p.m. to 6:45 a.m. Nine hours per night.

- A seventeen-year-old who goes to sleep around 1:00 a.m. and wakes at 7:00 a.m. is getting six hours and is missing at least two (for adequate sleep). His initial goal is to reach adequate sleep by moving his bedtime earlier by thirty minutes each week, until he's at 11:00 p.m. He will also keep to an 8:30 a.m. wake time on the weekend to reduce social jet lag.

HABIT #2: LAY OUT YOUR THREE ROUTINES

Write down your new wind-down, bedtime, and morning routine. Look at pages 158–163 for ideas. Remember to include both practical steps (like wash face and pack backpack) as well as enjoyable steps (like watch an episode of TV, read a graphic novel, or listen to a podcast).

Wind-down routine: _____

Bedtime routine: _____

Morning routine: _____

HABIT #3: EXTRACT YOUR SLEEP STEALERS

Look at the lists of unhelpful sleep associations and remove them. Remember these are anything that is happening *right before or as you fall asleep*. Some of the helpful sleep associations emerge naturally (like darkness and cool sheets), while others can be added actively (like passive distractions, page 169).

Check the box next to the association(s) you will eliminate.

Unhelpful sleep associations (what I'm doing right before or as I fall asleep):

- ☐ Interacting with phones, tablets, computers
- ☐ Texts, emails, video games, social media, talking on phone
- ☐ Watching television as I fall asleep

☐ News, alerts, stressful discussions

☐ Falling asleep on the couch or other location than bed

☐ Falling asleep with the lights on

☐ _____

☐ _____

☐ _____

Check the box next to the association(s) you will have/add.

Sleep-promoting associations (what I'm doing as I fall asleep):

☐ The feel of my blankets, pillows, and body position

☐ My dark, quiet bedroom

☐ Space in my mind, my own thoughts and imagery

☐ Trusting my body and letting go

☐ Simple meditation or relaxation breathing (see the appendix)

☐ Listening to an audiobook or podcast (see page 169)

☐ _____

☐ _____

☐ _____

HABIT #4: MAKE YOUR BEDROOM A CAVE

Create a dark, cool, quiet cave environment with the following checklists. This is a chance to design an enticing, sleep-welcoming bedroom that you look forward to nestling into.

Must-dos

These simple adjustments are basic to falling asleep easily, so it's best to put them in place right away (you'll see overlap between these and your wind-down and bedtime routines):

- Dim the light in your home one to two hours before bedtime.
- Put away phones, tablets, computers, and any close-held screens an hour before bedtime.
- Close blinds or curtains, preferably blackout.
- Turn off all lights, including any decorative lights or lamps, in your bedroom before climbing into bed.
- Lower thermostat to 65–68 degrees, thirty minutes before bedtime (or as cool as is reasonable in the summer).
- Make sure you have the right covers to be comfortable and cozy.

Can-dos

Enhance your dark, cool cave even more with these ideas or some of your own.

- Get a lower intensity light or "sleep friendly" book light for reading before bed.
- Be a light detective: make sure there are no other sources of light in your bedroom.
- Install dimmers on your wall switches and lamps.
- Order your blackout shades or curtain.
- Figure out how to dim your bathroom for showering, brushing teeth, and so forth before bed. A night-light is a good option in the bathroom.
- Set up a workspace and hangout space that is not your bed.
- Invest in a new set of sheets and pillow for your bed. If you make your bed feel special and super comfortable, you are more likely to look forward to slipping under the covers.
- Same goes for new pj's or a new nightgown. Make sure you have something you love to wear to bed.
- Wash your sheets once a week. Amazingly, people who wash their sheets weekly get more sleep. Have a second set of sheets on hand and make it a new habit.

- If you like strings of LED lights in your bedroom, choose warm colors like amber, red, and yellow and turn them off before you get into bed to journal or read.
- If you are especially sensitive to light before bed, find a lightbulb for your bedside table lamp that is designed to simulate sunset and promote falling asleep.
- If you like listening to soothing music, audiobooks, or podcasts, figure out how to do so without using a phone or tablet in bed, or at least to put "Do not disturb" on. If you have a smart speaker or an old-fashioned CD player, those will work. Be creative!
- If you live in a noisy home or neighborhood, try earplugs, a fan, or a sound machine to block noises.

HABIT #5: PRACTICE A SLEEP-FRIENDLY DAYTIME

Review the section (page 178) on ways to protect your sleep with your daytime habits. For each of these, make a note as to the changes or additions you will make.

1. Morning light _____

   Be outside for five to thirty minutes (depending on how sunny it is) when you first wake up in the morning, or as early as possible. This is also important on the weekends, to keep your internal clock in sync. Write down where you will do this and anything else about this morning ritual. (Eat breakfast, run around the block, take the dog for a walk...)

2. Exercise _____

   Regular, moderate exercise is good for sleep. Ideally, it should not be done too close to bedtime. Write down your exercise times and activities. See if there is any practice or exercise happening too late (and perhaps under bright lights).

3. Foods that support healthy sleep

Eat lots of vegetables, fruits, beans, nuts, seeds, and whole grains, while getting plenty of fiber and limiting sugar, refined carbs, and saturated fats.

- Foods I will eat more of _____

- Foods I will eat less of _____

- Caffeine cutoff time _____

Write down your cutoff time for caffeine and energy drinks. Everyone's a little different, but somewhere between 12:00 p.m. and 2:00 p.m. is a good cutoff time for most. This includes coffee, soda, caffeinated tea, and energy drinks. Remember that vaping products often have nicotine in them, which is a stimulant.

- Alcohol _____

Limit alcohol and avoid drinking it in the two hours before your bedtime.

- Bedtime snacks _____

If you like a bedtime snack, choose something small and that is easy to digest. Avoid spicy and fatty foods too close to bedtime, as well as big portions of any food. For example, a bowl of cereal and milk. Heather makes her family a plate of walnuts, crackers, cheese, and sliced fruit while they watch TV together before bed (her dad did the same for her as a kid).

4. Smart napping _____

If, after modifying your five habits, you are not able to sleep enough at night (for example, because of a too-early school start time and lots of homework), napping may be a good option for you. If you do nap, it's ideal to do it every day so it becomes routine, to nap in the afternoon, not in the evening, and to keep naps to about twenty to thirty minutes.

STEP 4: THE SLEEP CHALLENGE

Your challenge is to use the tools you've learned to reach the goal you wrote in Step 2. It often takes at least one week for your body to learn new timing and habits and to see an improvement in your sleep. For this reason, commit to a period of time in which to change your sleep habits, to allow your brain to learn these new patterns. We recommend choosing a seven-, fourteen-, or twenty-eight-day period in which you'll commit to your new habits. You can use the following table to make notes and track your progress. You will also find this at thehappysleeper.com.

Rewrite your goal from Step 2 here:

_____

NOTES	DAY	BEDTIME	WAKE-UP TIME	HOURS OF SLEEP
	Day 1			
	Day 2			
	Day 3			
	Day 4			
	Day 5			
	Day 6			
	Day 7			

NOTES	DAY	BEDTIME	WAKE-UP TIME	HOURS OF SLEEP

Here are some ideas for creating a challenge. Feel free to adjust them to what's best suited to you and your group or family:

- Teens can create a five-day challenge with a group of friends to do on weekdays.
- A sports team or theater group can do a challenge together as they prepare for a big game or performance. (Remember how LeBron loves sleep? So does Beyoncé.) See page 123 to lock your team in on the athletic benefits of more sleep. An actor will remember lines better with a good night's sleep before or after rehearsal. Sports coaches or directors, order each team or cast member a cozy sleep mask with the team's or play's name on it instead of swag T-shirts this year. Anything to inspire your teens and make it fun.
- The wonderful feeling of having slept well should be your main reward, but it can be fun to add in some lighthearted rewards for the person who "wins" the challenge. For example, if one person meets their goal after seven days, they are crowned "Sleep Champ" and they don't have to do dishes for the week. But who will win it the next week?

If you are taking the Sleep Challenge with a friend group or team, form a text group in which you report your hours of sleep or any other results every day or week. (No texting after wind-down time, though!) This will keep you accountable to each other and help you support each other. If you do the Sleep Challenge as a family, keep the mood light and curious. Everyone is on their own path. Note each person's progress toward more hours of sleep and which adjustments they were able to stick to. For those who made positive progress, discuss the changes to how they are feeling during the day and the benefits they're noticing. Let each person express their awareness of the connection between sleeping longer and feeling better on their own, rather than saying something like "Aren't you feeling better now?" If someone made little or no progress, that's okay too. Our lives and chemistries are not the same. Brainstorm tweaks to make that align better with your life. Just remember to gently go back to creating small, incremental, and achievable adjustments for the next week, and remember that small changes add up, gradually allowing you to hear your brain's and body's cues and to naturally fill up on healthy sleep.

Appendix

Sleep Meditations and Relaxation Tools
READY, SET, SLEEP?

S o, you've done your wind-down, followed your lovely bedtime routine, and made it under the covers by your new, regular bedtime in
your dark, cool bedroom. Hooray for you! But wait, you're lying
there wide awake and your thoughts are racing around in your mind.
Sleep eludes you.

Sometimes this happens because a text conversation, a game, or social
media you were just focusing on has wound you up into an agitated state.
Often, the cascading thoughts are everything on your "worry list" that you
managed to distract yourself from up to the moment of lying quietly in the
dark. Some of us get increasingly agitated, angry, and even fearful at the
thought that we might have a hard time falling asleep. As these thoughts
rush in, anxiety can increase and our outlook tends to be more negative.
We feel more vulnerable and our thoughts race around in our heads.

Buddhists refer to this as the "monkey mind"—a state of being un-
settled and restless. Sleep meditations and relaxation tools help you shut
down this activated state so your brain can let go and allow natural sleep

to take over. These tools shift your focus away from intrusive thoughts when you go to bed. They help you clear your mind, creating a more peaceful and spacious feeling. Think of it as changing the channel to one where you focus on sensations in your body and rhythms in your breath. By doing so, you bring yourself into the present moment rather than worrying about the past or future. These tools induce relaxation and calm your nervous system. Meditation aids sleep by reducing your heart rate, decreasing blood pressure, and increasing melatonin and serotonin, the sleepy hormones.

These tools are specifically designed for sleep (ideally, we stay awake when meditating during the day). Whichever one you choose, think of it as a practice rather than something you just do and see immediate results from. It helps to start slowly, with just three to five minutes each night. Be kind and patient with yourself, as it takes time, like training a muscle to become stronger.

MINDFULNESS MEDITATION

1. Lie down in your bed in your cool, dark, peaceful room. (Put on a sleep mask if you share a room or have any light in the room that you can't turn off.)
2. Move your attention to your breathing. Become aware of your breath and how it's cool as you inhale and warm as you exhale.
3. Slowly, begin to lengthen both your inhale and exhale without effort or strain.
4. Now count slowly to eight on your inhale, hold for four, and exhale for eight. Experiment with different counts that work best for you. Repeat five times or until you fall asleep.
5. When a thought comes up, gently send it away, knowing that you can revisit it the next day.

BODY SCAN MEDITATION

1. Lie down in your bed in your cool, dark, peaceful bedroom.
2. Close your eyes, slow your breath, and notice the weight of your body sinking into your mattress. Feel your body sink into your smooth sheets, cozy pillow, and comfortable bed.
3. Inhale slowly, and as you exhale, relax one part of your body. You can start with the top of your head or the tips of your toes. On each successive exhale, move your attention one body part at a time down or up your body, feeling it let go and drop down into your bed. Let gravity pull you gently down as you release. When you're done, you can reverse direction and continue.
4. If you reach a particularly tense spot, such as your eyes, jaw, neck, shoulders, chest, or stomach, stay with it, repeating step 3 until you feel it begin to soften and let go.
5. If you find your mind wandering, that's okay. Calmly bring your focus back to where you left off.

GUIDED MEDITATION OR IMAGERY

In guided meditation, you listen to a person's voice taking you through each step. This can include the two meditations above, breath focus and body scan, as well as guided imagery, storytelling, and visualizations. The choices for guided meditation are seemingly endless (see our website for ideas). Try out different choices to find the one that helps you quiet your thoughts and allows your body to pull you into sleep. Try a creative way to access these without having your phone beside you—like a smart speaker, an iPod, or an old-fashioned CD player if you can dig one out of the basement. If you listen on your phone, put it on "Do not disturb."

Guided meditations are probably so popular because, for some, they provide a stronger and more immediate distraction from our monkey minds. Some of our clients start out with guided meditation or imagery and then move to self-guided as their brains and bodies begin to habitually relax and let go more easily at bedtime. The benefit to the self-guided type is that you can access it at any time without technology.

Self-guided imagery: You are the sky

We love this self-guided meditation for its lovely simplicity, and so do many teens. It's based on a metaphor from Buddhist Pema Chödrön, who wrote,

You are the sky. Everything else—it's just the weather.

When our minds are caught up with all our personal worries and troubles, our focus narrows and our view becomes small. We tighten, contract, and get stuck in negativity and anxiety. We suffer, and needless to say, falling asleep becomes nearly impossible. This meditation allows us to step back and widen our perspective, opening up our mind's focus to the broad, expansive sky, seeing our thoughts and feelings as clouds or even storms that will pass by. We are the big broad sky and our stressful, overactive thoughts are the clouds. The consuming nature of our intrusive, anxiety-inducing thoughts becomes diluted and they lose their power against the massive sky.

You can use this mediation while you're riding to school in the morning, by looking up at the sky, or when you're walking home from school, as well as when you're falling asleep at night.

Day Sky Meditation: Look at the sky as you're walking or sitting outside, and imagine you are the whole expanse of blue—your whole life, including all the people in it, is a massive and magical, endless entity. Now see one of the clouds or overcast patches. This singular shape is whatever worry, fear, or trouble you're feeling. Imagine it's the heart-break, frustration, or fear—against the whole expanse of sky. It is there, but it is not you.

Night Sky Meditation: Lie comfortably in your bed. Close your eyes and slow your breathing. Imagine the beautiful blue sky all around you, as far as you can see. Say to yourself, "I am the sky." When negative, intrusive thoughts and feelings come into your mind, just think of them as clouds and watch them pass by; here one moment, gone the next. They come and they go, but they are not you. You are much more than them. They are just "the weather."

RELAXATION BREATHING

Relaxation breathing gets high marks for calming our nervous systems along with being easy to use. When we simply slow and lengthen our breathing, we send a message to our brain to calm down and relax. Our brain then sends this message to our body. The physical symptoms of stress and anxiety, such as increased heart rate, rapid breathing, and raised blood pressure, decrease as we begin to take long, deep breaths.

The type of relaxation breathing that is most effective in inducing these calming effects is often called "belly breathing."

1. Sit or lie flat in a comfortable position.
2. Put one hand over your belly button and the other hand on your chest.
3. Take a deep breath in through your nose, and let your belly push your hand out. Your chest should not move too much.
4. Breathe out through pursed lips as if you are whistling. Feel the hand on your belly go in, and use it to push all the air out.
5. Gradually slow and lengthen your breaths.

6. Some people like to count (work up to a count of eight on each inhale and exhale).

7. Do this breathing three to ten times. Take your time with each breath.

8. Notice how you feel at the end of the exercise.

WRITE DOWN YOUR WORRIES

Take a moment in the hour before bed to write down your top worries. Put your list in a drawer in a room other than your bedroom and promise yourself that it will be safe while you sleep and you can look at it in the morning. Say, "Bye-bye, list, see you in the morning!" It can help to say to yourself, "I can't do anything about these right now, but I can take some baby steps in the morning." There are different versions of this strategy. Some like to crumple up their list and throw it away, while others like to know that it's there for them to address at an appropriate time. Either way, this is a very effective pre-bedtime step that you can gently remind yourself about if and when the worries pop into your mind when you're trying to fall asleep.

THE 25-MINUTE RULE

If you find yourself wide awake about twenty-five minutes after going to bed or waking up during the night, the first time this happens, do nothing. Lie there in the dark (do not turn any lights on or check anything—make sure no clocks are facing you). Stay in the dark sleep cave you have created. Getting up can create a habit of, well, getting up—because your internal clock learns this and figures the next night it should wake you around this time too. Do nothing, remember it's normal to wake in the night, and trust that you will eventually fall back to sleep.

However, if you've practiced the five habits for a week or two and you're still finding yourself awake more than twenty-five minutes in bed, it's time to try something else. Get out of bed and occupy yourself with a calm, not-too-interesting activity until you start to feel sleepy. The reason for this is to avoid associating your bed with a place where you lie awake rather than a place where you sleep. You can go into the living room and, in dim light, read a book, stretch gently, listen to a podcast or audiobook, or do any non-screen activity that's not super activating or engaging. When you start to feel drowsy, climb back into bed.

AT THE END OF THE DAY

Stress and an overactive mind can often stand in the way of a good night's sleep. While these tools can be critical to helping you fall asleep, they don't replace the Five Habits of Happy Sleepers for creating your sleep bubble outlined in chapter 6. Think of them as the icing on your cake, but don't forget about your cake!

No matter which of these tools you choose, don't focus on "trying to sleep." Your overarching goal is to get out of your body's way and trust that it knows what to do. You can focus on what works best for you to feel soothed and safe in your bed, with a calm and spacious mind.

Notes

1. THE GREAT SLEEP RECESSION

Sleep levels in U.S. middle and high schools

National Sleep Foundation, *2006 Sleep in America*. National Sleep Foundation Poll. https://www.sleepfoundation.org/professionals/sleep-americar-polls/2006-teens -and-sleep.

U.S. measurements of adolescent sleep over the decades

Keyes, K. M., J. Maslowsky, A. Hamilton, and J. Schulenberg. "The Great Sleep Recession: Changes in Sleep Duration Among US Adolescents, 1991–2012." *Pediatrics* 135, no. 3 (2015): 460–68. doi: 10.1542/peds.2014-2707.

Tarokh, L., J. M. Saletin, and M. A. Carskadon. "Sleep in Adolescence: Physiology, Cognition and Mental Health." *Neuroscience and Biobehavioral Reviews* 70 (2016): 182–88. https://doi.org/10.1016/j.neubiorev.2016.08.008.

Twenge, J. M., Z. Krizan, and G. Hisler. "Decreases in Self-Reported Sleep Duration Among U.S. Adolescents 2009–2015 and Association with New Media Screen Time." *Sleep Medicine* 39 (2017): 47–53.

Sleep deprivation as a chronic stressor

McEwen, B. S. "Sleep Deprivation as a Neurobiologic and Physiologic Stressor: Allostasis and Allostatic Load." *Metabolism: Clinical and Experimental* 55, no. 10, suppl. 2 (2006): S20—S23.

Mental health and sleep

Centers for Disease Control and Prevention. *Youth Risk Behavior Survey: 2009–2019.* https://www.cdc.gov/healthyyouth/data/yrbs/yrbs_data_summary_and_trends.htm.

Fredriksen, K., J. Rhodes, R. Reddy, and N. Way. "Sleepless in Chicago: Tracking the Effects of Adolescent Sleep Loss During the Middle School Years." *Child Development* 75, no. 1 (2004): 84–95. doi: 10.1111/j.1467-8624.2004.00655.x.

Liu, X. "Sleep and Adolescent Suicidal Behavior." *Sleep* 27, no. 7 (2004): 1351–58.

National Vital Statistics Reports, U.S. Department of Health and Human Services, Centers for Disease Control and Prevention. "State Suicide Rates Among Adolescents and Young Adults Aged 10–24: United States 2000–2018." September 2020. https://stacks .cdc.gov/view/cdc/93667.

Whitmore, L. M., and T. C. Smith. "Isolating the Association of Sleep, Depressive State, and Other Independent Indicators for Suicide Ideation in United States Teenagers." *Archives of Suicide Research: Official Journal of the International Academy for Suicide Research* 23, no. 3 (2019): 471–490. doi: 10.1080/13811118.2018.1456992.

Sleep inequality

Curtis, D. S., T. E. Fuller-Rowell, M. El-Sheikh, M. R. Carnethon, and C. D. Ryff. "Habitual Sleep as a Contributor to Racial Differences in Cardiometabolic Risk." *Proceedings of the National Academy of Sciences of the USA* 114, no. 33 (2017): 8889–94. doi: 10.1073/pnas.1618167114.

Hale, L., W. Troxel, and D. J. Buysse. "Sleep Health: An Opportunity for Public Health to Address Health Equity." *Annual Review of Public Health* 41, no. 1 (2020): 81–99. doi: 10.1146/annurev-publhealth-040119-094412.

Marco, C. A., A. R. Wolfson, M. Sparling, and A. Azuaje. "Family Socioeconomic Status and Sleep Patterns of Young Adolescents." *Behavioral Sleep Medicine* 10, no. 1 (2011): 70–80. doi: 10.1080/15402002.2012.636298.

Risky behaviors and sleep

Centers for Disease Control and Prevention. *Teen Drivers: Get the Facts.* https://www.cdc.gov/motorvehiclesafety/teen_drivers/teendrivers_factsheet.html.

McKnight-Eily, L. R., et al. "Relationships Between Hours of Sleep and Health-Risk Behaviors in US Adolescent Students." *Preventive Medicine* 53, nos. 4–5 (2011): 271–73. doi: 10.1016/j.ypmed.2011.06.020.

Winsler, A., A. Deutsch, R. D. Vorona, P. A. Payne, and M. Szklo-Coxe. "Sleepless in Fairfax: The Difference One More Hour of Sleep Can Make for Teen Hopelessness, Suicidal Ideation, and Substance Use." *Journal of Youth and Adolescence* 44, no. 2 (2015): 362–78. doi: 10.1007/s10964-014-0170-3.

Academics and sleep

Gillen-O'Neel, C., V. W. Huynh, and A. J. Fuligni. "To Study or to Sleep? The Academic Costs of Extra Studying at the Expense of Sleep." *Child Development* 84, no. 1 (2013): 133–12. doi: 10.1111/j.1467-8624.2012.01834.x.

Adolescent sleep around the world

Gariepy, G., et al. "How Are Adolescents Sleeping? Adolescent Sleep Patterns and Sociodemographic Differences in 24 European and North American Countries." *Journal of Adolescent Health* 66, no. 6S (2020): S81—S88. doi: 10.1016/j.jadohealth.2020.03.013.

Loessl, B., et al. "Are Adolescents Chronically Sleep-Deprived? An Investigation of Sleep Habits of Adolescents in the Southwest of Germany." *Child: Care, Health and Development* 34, no. 5 (2008): 549–56. doi: 10.1111/j.1365-2214.2008.00845.x.

Ohida, T., et al. "An Epidemiologic Study of Self-Reported Sleep Problems Among Japanese Adolescents." *Sleep* 27, no. 5 (2004): 978–85. doi: 10.1093/sleep/27.5.978.

Olds, T., C. Maher, S. Blunden, and L. Matricciani. "Normative Data on the Sleep Habits of Australian Children and Adolescents." *Sleep* 33, no. 10 (2010): 1381–88. doi: 10.1093/sleep/33.10.1381.

Yang, C. K., J. K. Kim, S. R. Patel, and J. H. Lee. "Age-Related Changes in Sleep/Wake Patterns Among Korean Teenagers." *Pediatrics* 115, 1 suppl. (2005): 250–56. doi: 10.1542 /peds.2004-0815G.

Recognizing sleep issues

National Institute on Drug Abuse. *Monitoring the Future Study: Trends in Prevalence of Various Drugs for 8th Graders, 10th Graders, and 12th Graders* (2017–2020). https:// www.drugabuse.gov/drug-topics/trends-statistics/monitoring-future/monitoring -future-study-trends-in-prevalence-various-drugs.

National Sleep Foundation. *Communications Technology in the Bedroom.* 2011 Sleep in America poll. https://www.sleepfoundation.org/wp-content/uploads/2018/10 /SIAP_2011_Summary_of_Findings.pdf.

Short, M. A., M. Gradisar, J. Gill, and D. Camfferman. "Identifying Adolescent Sleep Problems." *PLoS One* 8, no. 9 (2013): e75301.

Earlier parent-set bedtimes and sleep

Gangwisch, J. E., et al. "Earlier Parental Set Bedtimes as a Protective Factor Against Depression and Suicidal Ideation." *Sleep* 33, no. 1 (2010): 97–106. doi: 10.1093 /sleep/33.1.97.

Athletes and sleep

Mah, C. D., K. E. Mah, E. J. Kezirian, and W. C. Dement. "The Effects of Sleep Extension on the Athletic Performance of Collegiate Basketball Players." *Sleep* 34, no. 7 (2011): 943–50. doi: 10.5665/SLEEP.1132.

Reyner, L. A., and J. A. Horne. "Sleep Restriction and Serving Accuracy in Performance Tennis Players, and Effects of Caffeine." *Physiology & Behavior* 120 (2013): 93–96. doi: 10.1016/j.physbeh.2013.07.002.

Schwartz, J., and R. D. Simon Jr. "Sleep Extension Improves Serving Accuracy: A Study with College Varsity Tennis Players." *Physiology & Behavior* 151 (2015): 541–44. doi: 10.1016/j.physbeh.2015.08.035.

Inspiration for our technology heading

Adachi-Mejia, A. M., P. M. Edwards, D. Gilbert-Diamond, G. P. Greenough, and A. L. Olson. "TXT Me I'm Only Sleeping: Adolescents with Mobile Phones in Their Bedroom." *Family & Community Health* 37, no. 4 (2014): 252–57. doi: 10.1097/FCH .0000000000000044.

2. THE ESSENTIAL NUTRIENT OF THE ADOLESCENT BRAIN
Brain changes and sleep

Bourgeois, J. P., and P. Rakic. "Changes of Synaptic Density in the Primary Visual Cortex of the Macaque Monkey from Fetal to Adult Stage." *Journal of Neuroscience* 13, no. 7 (1993): 2801–20. doi: 10.1523/JNEUROSCI.13-07-02801.1993.

Buchmann, A., et al. "EEG Sleep Slow-Wave Activity as a Mirror of Cortical Maturation." *Cerebral Cortex* 21, no. 3 (2011): 607–15. doi: 10.1093/cercor/bhq129.

Dahl, R. E., and M. El-Sheikh. "Considering Sleep in a Family Context: Introduction to the Special Issue." *Journal of Family Psychology* 21, no. 1 (2007): 1–3. doi: 10.1037/0893 -3200.21.1.1.

Frank, M. G., N. P. Issa, and M. P. Stryker. "Sleep Enhances Plasticity in the Developing Visual Cortex." *Neuron* 30, no. 1 (2001): 275–87. doi: 10.1016/s0896-6273(01)00279-3.

Galván, A. "The Need for Sleep in the Adolescent Brain. *Trends in Cognitive Sciences* 24, no. 1 (2020): 79–89. doi: 10.1016/j.tics.2019.11.002.

Hagenauer, M. H., and T. M. Lee. "Adolescent Sleep Patterns in Humans and Laboratory Animals." *Hormones and Behavior* 64, no. 2 (2013): 270–79. doi: 10.1016/j.yhbeh .2013.01.013.

Jalbrzikowski, M., et al. "Associations Between Brain Structure and Sleep Patterns Across Adolescent Development." *Sleep* 44, no. 10 (2021): zsab120. doi: 10.1093/sleep /zsab120.

Shaffery, J. P., J. Lopez, G. Bissette, and H. P. Roffwarg. "Rapid Eye Movement Sleep Deprivation in Post-Critical Period, Adolescent Rats Alters the Balance Between Inhibitory and Excitatory Mechanisms in Visual Cortex." *Neuroscience Letters* 393, nos. 2–3 (2006): 131–35. doi: 10.1016/j.neulet.20.09.051.

Tarokh, L., and M. A. Carskadon. "Developmental Changes in the Human Sleep EEG During Early Adolescence." *Sleep* 33, no. 6 (2010): 801–809. doi:10.1093/sleep/33.6.801.

Sleep and mental health

Balocchini, E., G. Chiamenti, and A. Lamborghini. "Adolescents: Which Risks for Their Life and Health?" *Journal of Preventive Medicine and Hygiene* 54, no. 4 (2013): 191–94. https://pubmed.ncbi.nlm.nih.gov/24779278/.

Gregory, A. M., F. V. Rijsdijk, J. Y. Lau, R. E. Dahl, and T. C. Eley. "The Direction of Longitudinal Associations Between Sleep Problems and Depression Symptoms: A Study of Twins Aged 8 and 10 Years." *Sleep* 32, no. 2 (2009): 189–99. doi: 10.1093/sleep/32.2.189.

Guzman-Marin, R., T. Bashir, N. Suntsova, R. Szymusiak, and D. McGinty. "Hippocampal Neurogenesis Is Reduced by Sleep Fragmentation in the Adult Rat." *Neuroscience* 148, no. 1 (2007): 325–33. doi: 10.1016/j.neuroscience.2007.05.030.

Harvard Health Publishing. "Sleep and Mental Health." August 17, 2021. https://www .health.harvard.edu/newsletter_article/sleep-and-mental-health.

Krause, A. J., et al. "The Sleep-Deprived Human Brain." *Nature Reviews Neuroscience* 18, no. 7 (2017): 404–18. doi: 10.1038/nrn.2017.55.

Talbot, L. S., E. L. McGlinchey, K. A. Kaplan, R. E. Dahl, and A. G. Harvey. "Sleep Deprivation in Adolescents and Adults: Changes in Affect." *Emotion* 10, no. 6 (2010): 831–41. doi: 10.1037/a0020138.

Yoo, S. S., N. Gujar, P. Hu, F. A. Jolesz, and M. P. Walker. "The Human Emotional Brain Without Sleep—A Prefrontal Amygdala Disconnect." *Current Biology* 17, no. 20 (2007): R877—R878. doi: 10.1016/.cub.2007.08.007.

Sleep and risky behaviors

Braams, B. R., A. C. van Duijvenvoorde, J. S. Peper, and E. A. Crone. "Longitudinal Changes in Adolescent Risk-Taking: A Comprehensive Study of Neural Responses to Rewards,

Pubertal Development, and Risk-Taking Behavior." *Journal of Neuroscience* 35, no. 18 (2015): 7226–38. doi: 10.1523/JNEUROSCI.4764-14.2015.

Chein, J., D. Albert, L. O'Brien, K. Uckert, and L. Steinberg. "Peers Increase Adolescent Risk Taking by Enhancing Activity in the Brain's Reward Circuitry." *Developmental Science* 14, no. 2 (2011): F1–F10. doi: 10.1111/j.1467-7687.2010.01035.x.

Guzman-Marin, R., T. Bashir, N. Suntsova, R. Szymusiak, and D. McGinty. "Hippocampal Neurogenesis Is Reduced by Sleep Fragmentation in the Adult Rat." *Neuroscience* 148, no. 1 (2007): 325–33. doi: 10.1016/j.neuroscience.2007.05.030.

Telzer, E. H., A. J. Fuligni, M. D. Lieberman, and A. Galván. "The Effects of Poor Quality Sleep on Brain Function and Risk Taking in Adolescence." *NeuroImage* 71 (2013): 275–83. doi: 10.1016/j.neuroimage.2013.01.025.

Weaver, M. D., L. K. Barger, S. K. Malone, L. S. Anderson, and E. B. Klerman. "Dose-Dependent Associations Between Sleep Duration and Unsafe Behaviors Among US High School Students." *JAMA Pediatrics* 172, no. 12 (2018): 1187–89. doi: 10.1001/jama pediatrics.2018.2777.

3. ADOLESCENT SLEEP

Classic studies on adolescent sleep

Carskadon, M. A., et al. "Pubertal Changes in Daytime Sleepiness." *Sleep* 2, no. 4 (1980): 453–60. doi: 10.1093/sleep/2.4.453.

Carskadon, M. A., A. R. Wolfson, C. Acebo, O. Tzischinsky, and R. Seifer. "Adolescent Sleep Patterns, Circadian Timing, and Sleepiness at a Transition to Early School Days." *Sleep* 21, no. 8 (1998): 871–81. doi: 10.1093/sleep/21.8.871.

Dement, W. C. *The Promise of Sleep*. New York: Dell, 2000.

The "perfect storm"

Carskadon, M. A. "Sleep in Adolescents: The Perfect Storm." *Pediatric Clinics of North America* 58, no. 3 (2011): 637–47. doi: 10.1016/j.pcl.2011.03.003.

Crowley, S. J., A. R. Wolfson, L. Tarokh, and M. A. Carskadon. "An Update on Adolescent Sleep: New Evidence Informing the Perfect Storm Model." *Journal of Adolescence* 67 (2018): 55–65. doi: 10.1016/j.adolescence.2018.06.001.

Further studies of adolescent sleep needs and patterns

Carskadon, M. A., C. Acebo, and R. Seifer. "Extended Nights, Sleep Loss, and Recovery Sleep in Adolescents." *Archives Italiennes de Biologie* 139, no. 3 (2001): 301–12.

Challenge Success and NBC News. *Kids Under Pressure: A Look at Student Well-Being and Engagement During the Pandemic*. February 2021. https://challengesuccess.org /wp-content/uploads/2021/02/CS-NBC-Study-Kids-Under-Pressure-PUBLISHED.pdf.

Fuligni, A. J., S. Bai, J. L. Krull, and N. A. Gonzales. "Individual Differences in Optimum Sleep for Daily Mood During Adolescence." *Journal of Clinical Child & Adolescent Psychology* 48, no. 3 (2019): 469–79. doi: 10.1080/15374416.2017.1357126.

Jones, J. M. "In U.S., 40% Get Less Than Recommended Amount of Sleep." Gallup, December 13, 2019. https://news.gallup.com/poll/166553/less-recommended-amount-sleep .aspx.

Keyes, K. M., J. Maslowsky, A. Hamilton, and J. Schulenberg. "The Great Sleep Recession: Changes in Sleep Duration Among US Adolescents, 1991–2012." *Pediatrics* 135, no. 3 (2015): 460–68. doi: 10.1542/peds.2014-2707.

National Sleep Foundation, *2006 Sleep in America*. National Sleep Foundation Poll. https://www.sleepfoundation.org/professionals/sleep-americar-polls/2006-teens -and-sleep.

Changes in the adolescent sleep clock
Crowley, S. J., S. W. Cain, A. C. Burns, C. Acebo, and M. A. Carskadon. "Increased Sensitivity of the Circadian System to Light in Early/Mid-Puberty." *Journal of Clinical Endocrinology & Metabolism* 100, no. 11 (2015): 4067–73. doi: 10.1210/jc.2015-2775.

Hagenauer, M. H., J. I. Perryman, T. M. Lee, and M. A. Carskadon. "Adolescent Changes in the Homeostatic and Circadian Regulation of Sleep." *Developmental Neuroscience* 31, no. 4 (2009): 276–84. doi: 10.1159/000216538.

Optimal versus adequate sleep
McKnight-Eily, L. R., et al. "Relationships Between Hours of Sleep and Health-Risk Behaviors in US Adolescent Students." *Preventive Medicine* 53, nos. 4–5 (2011): 271–73. doi: 10.1016/j.ypmed.2011.06.020.

Nature, camping, and access to lights
de la Iglesia, H. O., et al. "Access to Electric Light Is Associated with Shorter Sleep Duration in a Traditionally Hunter-Gatherer Community." *Journal of Biological Rhythms* 30, no. 4 (2015): 342–50. doi: 10.1177/0748730415590702.

Stothard, E. R., et al. "Circadian Entrainment to the Natural Light-Dark Cycle Across Seasons and the Weekend." *Current Biology* 27, no. 4 (2017): 508–513. doi: 10.1016/j .cub.2016.12.041.

Jet lag
Ben-Hamo, M., et al. "Circadian Forced Desynchrony of the Master Clock Leads to Phenotypic Manifestation of Depression in Rats." *eNeuro* 3, no. 6 (2017): ENEURO.0237 -16.2016.

Regularity is just as important as how much
Fang, Y., D. B. Forger, E. Frank, S. Sen, and C. Goldstein. "Day-to-Day Variability in Sleep Parameters and Depression Risk: a Prospective Cohort Study of Training Physicians." *npj Digital Medicine* 4 (2021): article no. 28.

Disruption of circadian clock in mice
Karatsoreos, I. N., S. Bhagat, E. B. Bloss, J. H. Morrison, and B. S. McEwen. "Disruption of Circadian Clocks Has Ramifications for Metabolism, Brain, and Behavior." *Proceedings of the National Academy of Sciences of the USA* 108, no. 4 (2011): 1657–62. doi: 10.1073/pnas.1018375108.

Afternoon classes result in reduced jet lag and more sleep

Carvalho-Mendes, R. P., G. P. Dunster, H. O. de la Iglesia, and L. Menna-Barreto. "Afternoon School Start Times Are Associated with a Lack of Both Social Jetlag and Sleep Deprivation in Adolescents." *Journal of Biological Rhythms* 35, no. 4 (2020): 377–90. doi: 10.1177/0748730420927603.

Social jet lag and obesity

Roenneberg, T., K. V. Allebrandt, M. Merrow, and C. Vetter. "Social Jetlag and Obesity." *Current Biology* 22, no. 10 (2012): 939–43. doi: 10.1016/j.cub.2012.03.038.

Teen sleep needs and risk

Colrain, I. M., and F. C. Baker. "Changes in Sleep as a Function of Adolescent Development." *Neuropsychology Review* 21, no. 1 (2011): 5–21. doi: 10.1007/s11065-010-9155-5.

Pandemic sleep

Wright, K. P., et al. "Sleep in University Students Prior to and During COVID-19 Stay-at-Home Orders." *Current Biology* 30, no. 14 (2020): R797—R798. doi: 10.1016/j.cub.2020.06.022.

4. SCREENS, TEENS, AND THE MISSING LINK
Relationship between screen time and mental health

Liu, S., et al. "The Associations of Long-Time Mobile Phone Use with Sleep Disturbances and Mental Distress in Technical College Students: A Prospective Cohort Study." *Sleep* 42, no. 2 (2019): zsy213. doi: 10.1093/sleep/zsy213.

Twenge, J. M., T. E. Joiner, M. L. Rogers, and G. N. Martin. "Increases in Depressive Symptoms, Suicide-Related Outcomes, and Suicide Rates Among U.S. Adolescents After 2010 and Links to Increased New Media Screen Time." *Clinical Psychological Science* 6, no. 1 (2018): 3–17. doi: 10.1177/2167702617723376.

Twenge, J. M., G. N. Martin, and W. K. Campbell. "Decreases in Psychological Well-Being Among American Adolescents After 2012 and Links to Screen Time During the Rise of Smartphone Technology." *Emotion* 18, no. 6 (2018): 765–80. doi: 10.1037/emo0000403.

Royal Society for Public Health. "#StatusofMind," May 2017. https://www.rsph.org.uk/our-work/campaigns/status-of-mind.html.

Screens and sleep

Bartel, K., R. Scheeren, and M. Gradisar. "Altering Adolescents' Pre-Bedtime Phone Use to Achieve Better Sleep Health." *Journal of Health Communication* 34, no. 4 (2019): 456–62. doi: 10.1080/10410236.2017.1422099.

Cajochen, C., et al. "Evening Exposure to a Light-Emitting Diodes (LED)–Backlit Computer Screen Affects Circadian Physiology and Cognitive Performance." *Journal of Applied Physiology* 110, no. 5 (2011): 1432–38. doi: 10.1152/japplphysiol.00165.2011.

Carter, B., P. Rees, L. Hale, D. Bhattacharjee, and M. S. Paradkar. "Association Between Portable Screen-Based Media Device Access or Use and Sleep Outcomes: A Systematic Review and Meta-Analysis." *JAMA Pediatrics* 170, no. 12 (2016): 1202–208. doi: 10.1001/jamapediatrics.2016.2341.

Leonard, H., A. Khurana, and M. Hammond. "Bedtime Media Use and Sleep: Evidence for Bidirectional Effects and Associations with Attention Control in Adolescents." *Sleep Health* 7, no. 4 (2021): 491–99. doi: 10.1016/j.sleh.2021.05.003.

Twenge, J. M., Z. Krizan, and G. Hisler. "Decreases in Self-Reported Sleep Duration Among U.S. Adolescents 2009–2015 and Association with New Media Screen Time." *Sleep Medicine* 39 (2017): 47–53. doi: 10.1016/j.sleep.2017.08.013.

Van der Lely, S., et al. "Blue Blocker Glasses as a Countermeasure for Alerting Effects of Evening Light-Emitting Diode Screen Exposure in Male Teenagers." *Journal of Adolescent Health* 56, no. 1 (2015): 113–19. doi: 10.1016/j.jadohealth.2014.08.002.

Italian study during COVID-19

Robb, M. B. *The New Normal: Parents, Teens, Screens, and Sleep in the United States*. San Francisco: Common Sense Media, 2019. https://www.commonsensemedia.org/sites/default/files/uploads/research/2019-new-normal-parents-teens-screens-and-sleep-united-states.pdf.

Salfi, F., et al. "Changes of Evening Exposure to Electronic Devices During the COVID-19 Lockdown Affect the Time Course of Sleep Disturbances." *Sleep* 44, no. 9 (2021): zsab080. doi: 10.1093/sleep/zsab080.

Babies and young kids, screens, and sleep

Garrison, M. M., K. Liekweg, and D. A. Christakis. "Media Use and Child Sleep: The Impact of Content, Timing, and Environment." *Pediatrics* 128, no. 1 (2011): 29–35. doi: 10.1542/peds.2010-3304.

Vijakkhana, N., T. Wilaisakditipakorn, K. Ruedeekhajorn, C. Pruksananonda, and W. Chonchaiya. "Evening Media Exposure Reduces Night-Time Sleep." *Acta Paediatrica* 104, no. 3 (2015): 306–12. doi: 10.1111/apa.12904.

COVID and physical activity

Schmidt, S., et al. "Physical Activity and Screen Time of Children and Adolescents Before and During the COVID-19 Lockdown in Germany: A Natural Experiment." *Scientific Reports* 10 (2020): article no. 21780. doi: 10.1038/s41598-02078438-4.

5. EARLY START TIMES AND ACADEMIC OVERLOAD

Testimonies before the school board and personal stories from Fairfax County parents and students can be found at http://www.sleepinfairfax.org/stories.htm.

Winsler, A., A. Deutsch, R. D. Vorona, P. A. Payne, and M. Szklo-Coxe. "Sleepless in Fairfax: The Difference One More Hour of Sleep Can Make for Teen Hopelessness, Suicidal Ideation, and Substance Use." *Journal of Youth and Adolescence* 44, no. 2 (2015): 362–78. doi: 10.1007/s10964-014-0170-3.

Commuting to school

Voulgaris, C. T., M. J. Smart, and B. Taylor. "Tired of Commuting? Relationships Among Journeys to School, Sleep, and Exercise Among American Teenagers." *Journal of Planning Education and Research* 39 (2017): 142–154.

Later start time studies

Carskadon, M. A., A. R. Wolfson, C. Acebo, O. Tzischinsky, and R. Seifer. "Adolescent Sleep Patterns, Circadian Timing, and Sleepiness at a Transition to Early School Days." *Sleep* 21, no. 8 (1998): 871–81. https://doi.org/10.1093/sleep/21.8.871.

Dunster, G. P., S. J. Crowley, M. A. Carskadon, and H. O. de la Iglesia. "What Time Should Middle and High School Students Start School?" *Journal of Biological Rhythms* 34, no. 6 (2019): 576–78. doi: 10.1177/0748730419892118.

Wahlstrom, K. "Changing Times: Findings from the First Longitudinal Study of Later High School Start Times." *NASSP Bulletin* 86, no. 633 (2002): 3–21. doi: 10.1177/019263650208663302.

Wahlstrom, K. L., et al. *Examining the Impact of Later School Start Times on the Health and Academic Performance of High School Students: A Multi-Site Study.* Center for Applied Research and Educational Improvement, University of Minnesota, 2014. https://www.spps.org/cms/lib010/MN01910242/Centricity/Domain/7352/final_version_3-11-14_start_time_report.pdf.

Widome, R., et al. "Association of Delaying School Start Time with Sleep Duration, Timing, and Quality Among Adolescents." *JAMA Pediatrics* 174, no. 7 (2020): 697–704. doi: 10.1001/jamapediatrics.2020.0344.

Driving and sleep

Bin-Hasan, S., K. Kapur, K. Rakesh, and J. Owens. "School Start Time Change and Motor Vehicle Crashes in Adolescent Drivers." *Journal of Clinical Sleep Medicine* 16, no. 3 (2020): 371–76.

Mawson, A. R., and E. K. Walley. "Toward an Effective Long-Term Strategy for Preventing Motor Vehicle Crashes and Injuries." *International Journal of Environmental Research and Public Health* 11, no. 8 (2014): 8123–36. doi: 10.3390/ijerph110808123.

Vorona, R. D., et al. "Dissimilar Teen Crash Rates in Two Neighboring Southeastern Virginia Cities with Different High School Start Times." *Journal of Clinical Sleep Medicine* 7, no. 2 (2011): 145–51.

Wahlstrom, K. L., et al. *Examining the Impact of Later School Start Times on the Health and Academic Performance of High School Students: A Multi-Site Study.* Center for Applied Research and Educational Improvement, University of Minnesota, 2014. https://www.spps.org/cms/lib010/MN01910242/Centricity/Domain/7352/final_version_3-11-14_start_time_report.pdf.

Grades, learning, and sleep alertness, learning and time of day

Galloway, M., J. Conner, and D. Pope. "Nonacademic Effects of Homework in Privileged, High-Performing High Schools." *Journal of Experimental Education* 81, no. 4 (2013): 490–510. doi: 10.1080/00220973.2012.745469.

Lo, J. C., J. L. Ong, R. L. Leong, J. J. Gooley, and M. W. Chee. "Cognitive Performance, Sleepiness, and Mood in Partially Sleep Deprived Adolescents: The Need for Sleep Study." *Sleep* 39, no. 3 (2016): 687–98. doi: 10.5665/sleep.5552.

Lufi, D., O. Tzischinsky, and S. Hadar. "Delaying School Starting Time by One Hour: Some Effects on Attention Levels in Adolescents." *Journal of Clinical Sleep Medicine* 7, no. 2 (2011): 137–43.

Wolfson, A. R., and M. A. Carskadon. "Sleep Schedules and Daytime Functioning in Adolescents." *Child Development* 69, no. 4 (1998): 875–87.

Wolfson, A. R., and M. A. Carskadon. "Understanding Adolescents' Sleep Patterns and School Performance: A Critical Appraisal." *Sleep Medicine Reviews* 7, no. 6 (2003): 491–506. doi: 10.1016/s1087-0792(03)90003-7.

Elementary schoolers

Meltzer, L. J., K. L. Wahlstrom, A. E. Plog, and M. J. Strand. "Changing School Start Times: Impact on Sleep in Primary and Secondary School Students." *Sleep* 44, no. 7 (2021): zsab048. doi: 10.1093/sleep/zsab048.

Economic and social benefits of later starts

Hafner, M., M. Stepanek, and W. M. Troxel. "Later School Start Times in the U.S.: An Economic Analysis." RAND Corporation, Santa Monica, California, 2017. https://www.rand.org/pubs/research_reports/RR2109.html.

Jacob, B. A., and J. E. Rockoff. *Organizing Schools to Improve Student Achievement: Start Times, Grade Configurations, and Teacher Assignments.* Brookings Institution, September 27, 2011.

Wolfson, A. R., and M. A. Carskadon. "A Survey of Factors Influencing High School Start Times." *NASSP Bulletin* 89, no. 642 (2005): 47–66. doi: 10.1177/019263650508964205.

Short sleep and napping

Lo, J. C., et al. "Neurobehavioral Impact of Successive Cycles of Sleep Restriction With and Without Naps in Adolescents." *Sleep* 40, no. 2 (2017): zsw042. https://doi.org/10.1093/sleep/zsw042.

Dikker, S., et al. "Morning Brain: Real-World Neural Evidence That High School Class Times Matter." *Social Cognitive and Affective Neuroscience* 15, no. 11 (2020): 1193–202. doi: 10.1093/scan/nsaa142.

Significantly later start times and impact

Kelley, P., S. W. Lockley, J. Kelley, and M. Evans. "Is 8:30 a.m. Still Too Early to Start School? A 10:00 a.m. School Start Time Improves Health and Performance of Students Aged 13–16." *Frontiers in Human Neuroscience* 11 (2017): 588. doi: 10.3389/fnhum.2017.00588.

Acknowledgments

We'd like to thank our editor, Sara Carder, for being a champion of this book right from the start, and for her amazing collaborative spirit and guidance through all the steps that have followed. Thank you to Ashley Alliano for her kindness, diligence, and hand-holding. And our agent, Michelle Tessler, for her steady and decisive voice, insight, and encouragement.

The scientists and experts who gave their feedback and ideas have been essential and we are so grateful for their time and careful consideration: Mary Carskadon, Horacio de la Iglesia, Maira Karan, and Dolly Klock. A special thanks to the amazing professional skill of Lisa Sweetingham, and to Phillis Payne of Start School Later, for her time, expertise, and dedication to teen sleep. Thank you to the parents, family, and friends who read this book, shared insights, and weighed in on creative aspects: Laurel Garber, Toby Huttner, Brynn Karwas, Alexis Landau, Lenna Lebovich, Suzy Manning, Mary Posatko, Rana Shanawani, Stacy Simera, Lisa Steele, Gillian Turgeon, and Robert Turgeon.

From Heather:

Writing a book is made possible by the love and enthusiasm of family and friends—and I am overflowing in that department. To my parents: Thank you for supporting me in everything I do, and for teaching me to write and to love science. You are my number one inspiration. As a teen, you set the bar high but kept the stress low (and you also helped me get to bed on time!). My extraordinary mom's group for their care and comic relief I wouldn't have survived the last two (actually, thirteen) years without. To Ben: Thank you for casting a creative magic on our work, and for believing in me so much that you never (ever) stop advocating for the best and helping me get there. I love you. To Dashiell and Eloise: I am the luckiest person in the whole world to be your mom. Thank you for your great ideas, humor, and enthusiasm for my work. You are everything.

From Julie:

I have to pinch myself in amazement when I think of the bounty of love and support in my life. Mom, you are my guiding light and my inspiration for helping others and following science. My dad, who died seventeen years ago, lives on within me, lending curiosity, outside-the-box thinking, and humor to my work. Jack, my dear son, with your steady love and kind soul, you uplift and delight me more than you'll ever know. To my beloved siblings, Susan, David, and Stephen, and your precious spouses, Phil, Sue, and Karen, along with my nieces, nephews, treasured friends, and colleagues, you are my village and my support system, always there to love and encourage me.

Index